ABC OF EMERGENCY RADIOLOGY

ABC OF EMERGENCY RADIOLOGY

edited by

DAVID A NICHOLSON, FRCR

Consultant radiologist, Hope Hospital, Salford

and

PETER A DRISCOLL, FRCS

Senior lecturer in accident and emergency medicine, Hope Hospital, Salford

with contributions by

W St C FORBES, D W HODGKINSON, P HUGHES, N KURDY, I LANG, R E LLOYD,
D MARSH, B R O'DRISCOLL, D O'KEEFFE, R ROSS, P SANVILLE, R TOUQUET

BMJ
Publishing
Group

© BMJ Publishing Group 1995

First published 1995
Reprinted 1996
Reprinted 1997
Reprinted 1998

British Library Cataloguing in Publication Data

A catalogue record for this book is available from the British Library

ISBN 0–7279–0832–4

Printed in the United Kingdom
at the University Press, Cambridge

Contents

FOREWORD

Radiography is expensive and x rays are potentially hazardous. Emergency medicine often bring together critically ill patients and relatively junior and inexperienced staff in an unstructured environment. This provides opportunities for inappropriate management, wasted resources, and unnecessary exposure of patients and staff to ionising radiation.

The *ABC of Emergency Radiology* is a most welcome initiative, epitomising the increasingly close collaboration between these two disciplines. The authors have a wealth of experience in the indications for, and interpretation of, radiographs that are ordered commonly in emergency situations.

The book is divided into fourteen chapters according to anatomical site. Each begins with a review of the normal radiological anatomy and includes normal variants that may be mistaken for traumatic lesions. Subsequently the important radiological abnormalities associated with trauma, and their clinical relevance are described.

The book is concerned primarily with teaching a systematic approach to basic radiographic interpretation, with emphasis on avoiding pitfalls in diagnosis. To ensure that the radiological examination performed is appropriate to the clinical situation it is helpful if guidelines of good practice, such as those produced by the Royal College of Radiologists in 1993, *Making the Best Use of a Department of Clinical Radiology*, be used in conjunction with the *ABC of Emergency Radiology*. Indeed it would be a short step to produce comprehensive management protocols based on the diagnostic criteria provided in the text.

Reproducing radiographs is always hazardous, but the publishers have succeeded in providing good quality films matched to excellent line diagrams. This book will prove invaluable in guiding recently qualified medical staff who either work in, or are called to, an accident and emergency department. It will also be of interest to GPs, nurses, and radiographers who are becoming involved increasingly in the requesting and interpretation of radiographs.

We are certain that this book will serve to raise the standards and confidence of those required to interpret radiographs in the acutely ill or traumatised patient and contribute to improved clinical management and appropriate use of resources and radiation dose.

PROFESSOR JUDITH ADAMS
Department of Diagnostic Radiology
PROFESSOR DAVID YATES
Department of Emergency Medicine
University of Manchester

INTRODUCTION

It is easy for clinicians to make mistakes when interpreting emergency radiographs because very few receive any formal training in this discipline. The situation is often made even more difficult by the urgency and circumstances in which the radiograph has to be evaluated. If an adequate history is taken, and the patient's physical signs assessed, all doctors should be able to correctly interpret the radiograph with the appropriate radiological knowledge. To interpret radiographs consistently and accurately doctors must be able to recognise when radiographs are not of diagnostic quality and follow a systematic, stepwise approach to the assessment of each radiograph.

This book aims to help doctors by describing a systematic approach to interpreting plain radiographs. This is augmented by illustrated algorithms, descriptions of the relevant anatomy, and, where appropriate, the common mechanisms of injury. Repeated use of this ordered radiological search will help establish a knowledge of normal appearances and should ultimately improve management of patients.

We thank Mary Harrison for preparing the line drawings.

D A NICHOLSON
P A DRISCOLL

Hope Hospital,
Salford

March 1994

HAND

D W Hodgkinson, N Kurdy, D A Nicholson, P A Driscoll

Injuries to the hand and wrist account for about 15% of attendances at accident and emergency departments. The hand and wrist are complex structures and injury to just one small component can result in appreciable loss of function. Fortunately if the injury is identified early and managed appropriately function can be fully restored.

Important anatomy

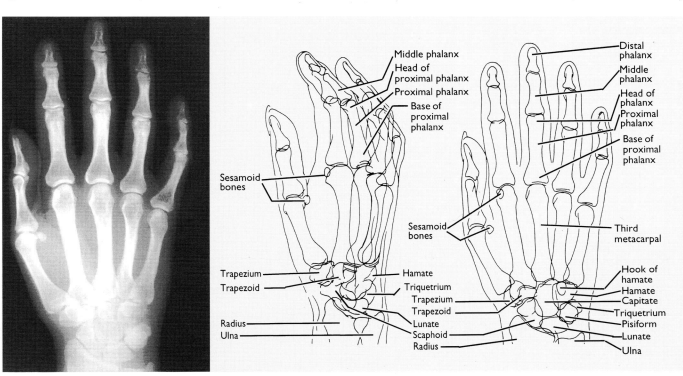

FIG 1—Posteroanterior radiograph and line drawing of normal hand.

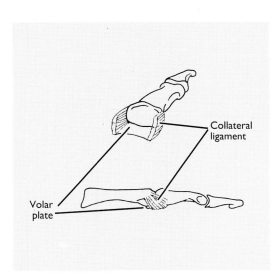

FIG 2—Collateral ligaments and volar plate of the proximal interphalangeal joint.

The 14 phalanges and five metacarpals in each hand consist of a head, a body, and a base. Collateral ligaments extend from the lateral margins of the head of each metacarpal bone and phalanx (except the terminal phalanx) across the appropriate joint space to insert on the lateral margin of the base of the apposing phalanx. The volar aspect of the interphalangeal and metacarpophalangeal joint capsule is thickened and forms a dense fibrous structure called the volar plate. Sesamoid bones may be found on the palmar surface of the hand. The two commonest are in the tendons of the thumb in the two heads of the flexor pollicis brevis at the metacarpophalangeal joint (fig 1). The other sesamoid bones of the hand are usually found at the metacarpophalangeal portion of the volar plate. Sideways movement of the thumb metacarpophalangeal joint is prevented by strong ulnar and radial collateral ligaments (fig 9).

Development

Secondary ossification centres (epiphyses) in the metacarpals and phalanges of the hand appear at the age of 2-3 years, and the growth plate normally closes at puberty. Skeletal age up to puberty can be judged accurately from hand and wrist radiographs as the sequence of development is age specific.

Mechanism of common injuries

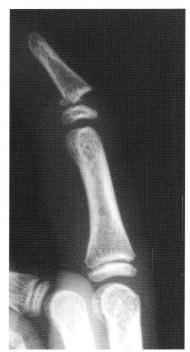

FIG 3—Lateral radiograph of a child's finger showing a type II Salter-Harris epiphyseal injury. There is dorsal displacement of the distal phalanx, and the injury is potentially unstable.

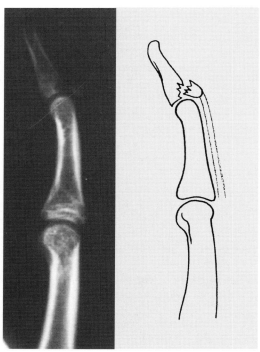

FIG 4—Lateral radiograph of a mallet finger with an avulsion fracture.

Finger tip injuries

These are commonly produced by a crush injury and may be associated with severe trauma to the soft tissue (including the nail bed and pulp) even if there is no bone injury. Fractures of the distal phalanx in adults and distal phalanx epiphysis in children may be compound into the nail bed. Distal phalanx epiphyseal injuries in children usually displace dorsally affecting the nail bed, and are potentially unstable (fig 3).

Mallet finger

This injury usually results from a direct blow to the extended digit—for example, a blow to the finger tip with a cricket ball. The mallet deformity is produced by avulsion of the extensor tendon from its insertion (not visible on radiography) or by an avulsion fracture at the base of the distal phalanx. Radiography is required to identify a fracture. If the fracture affects more than one third of the joint articular surface the joint may become unstable (fig 4).

Interphalangeal joint dislocation

This dislocation most commonly affects the proximal interphalangeal joint and is the result of a sporting injury. The volar plate tears or detaches at one end and the distal phalanx usually dislocates dorsally. A joint dislocation may be suspected on the posteroanterior view when the joint space is narrowed or incongruous (fig 5). The diagnosis must be confirmed with the lateral view. In most cases reduction is simple, but occasionally the torn volar plate or other soft tissues become interposed between the joint surfaces and prevent reduction. Radiographs taken after reduction should therefore be checked for possible missed fracture and for perfect joint congruity. Lack of congruity suggests interposition of soft tissue in the joint.

Avulsion fractures

These are flakes of bone pulled off at the attachments of the ligaments, capsule, or flexor and extensor tendons. They are common and should be suspected from the mechanism of injury and clinical findings. Avulsion flakes can be difficult to show radiologically as they may be visible in only one radiographic projection. The fracture can appear simple, but the underlying soft tissue injury may be serious. The soft tissue swelling visible in the radiograph may be the only indicator of injury.

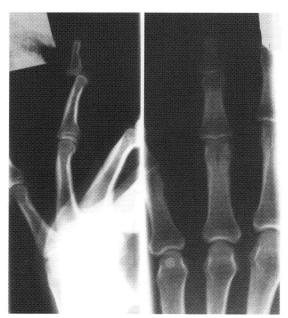

FIG 5—Distal interphalangeal joint dislocation. The lateral view (left) clearly shows the dislocation but it could be missed in the posteroanterior view (right) unless joint congruity is carefully checked.

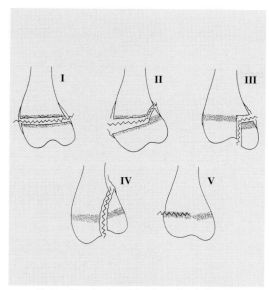

FIG 6—Salter-Harris classification of epiphyseal fractures.

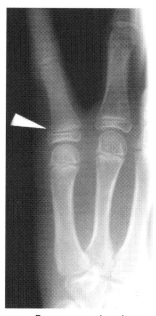

FIG 7—Posteroanterior view of the little finger showing a Salter-Harris type II injury to the base of the proximal phalanx (arrow).

Phalangeal and metacarpal shaft fractures

The mechanism of injury varies. Transverse and comminuted fractures reflect direct and possibly high energy trauma while spiral fractures are invariably produced by a rotational force. If a fracture is present always check for clinical evidence of rotational deformity in the finger. Radiological evidence of deformity can be misleading. Oblique radiographs show the metacarpals and phalanges separately. The oblique view is taken at 45° to the plane of the posteroanterior radiograph. They should be used for the assessment of these injuries. In the lateral view, which is exactly 90° to the plane of the posteroanterior radiograph, the metacarpals are superimposed, and this may result in misinterpretation.

Transverse fracture at the base of the proximal phalanx

This fracture is usually the result of hyperextension of the finger at the metacarpophalangeal joint. Severe dorsal angulation may be present and this can be underestimated clinically and radiologically. An oblique view should be used to assess the injury.

A Salter-Harris type II epiphyseal fracture of the base of the proximal phalanx of the little finger is common in children and results from an abduction force to the finger (figs 6 and 7). Ulnar angulation at the fracture site can be seen in the posteroanterior radiograph.

Boxer's fracture

Fracture of the metacarpal neck with volar displacement of the head usually occurs in the fifth metacarpal bone but it can occur less commonly in the other finger metacarpals (fig 8). It is normally due to a punch. Lateral and oblique views are required to identify any angulation. Associated wounds to the skin must be taken seriously since they may communicate directly with the metacarpophalangeal joint (particularly after delivering a blow to teeth).

Skier's (gamekeeper's) thumb

This is an acute sprain or rupture of the ulnar collateral ligament at the metacarpophalangeal joint caused by forceful abduction of the thumb (fig 9). The diagnosis is based on the history and clinical findings. Radiographs can appear normal or show only soft tissue swelling. Occasionally an avulsion fracture may be present.

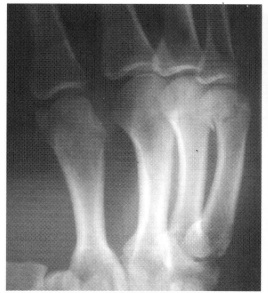
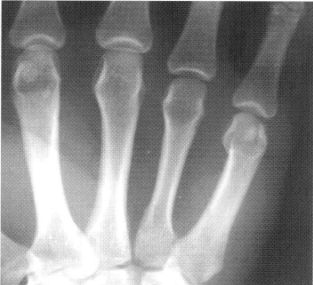

FIG 8—Posteroanterior and oblique view showing a moderately displaced boxer's fracture.

Hand

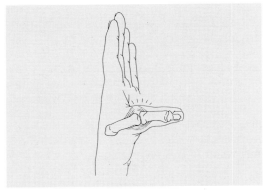

FIG 9—Mechanism of injury in rupture of the ulnar collateral ligament of the thumb metacarpophalangeal joint. There may be an avulsion fracture that can be seen in the plain radiograph; the orientation of the ligament and the adductor aponeurosis may be identifiable.

Bennett's fracture

This is a fracture dislocation of the thumb carpometacarpal joint. It usually results from forced abduction of the thumb. It is unstable because of the pull of the abductor pollicis longus tendon, which inserts into the base of the thumb metacarpal bone (fig 10).

Contusions, lacerations, and soft tissue injuries

The hand is often exposed to minor contusions and lacerations. The history and mechanism of injury will indicate the likelihood of a retained foreign body and the need for radiographic examination. Proper clinical assessment of the wound is essential even if the radiograph appears normal as many retained foreign bodies are radiolucent. Some soft tissue injuries are extremely disabling but produce few radiological abnormalities—for example, pneumatic and high pressure jet injuries. These should be identified from the history.

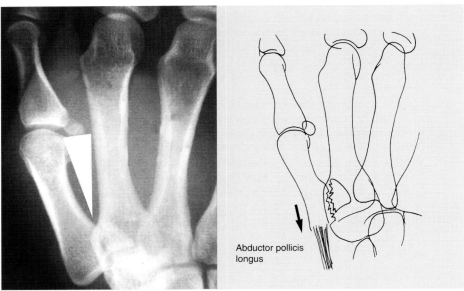

Abductor pollicis longus

FIG 10—Posteroanterior view and line drawing showing a Bennett's fracture dislocation (arrow).

Radiographic views

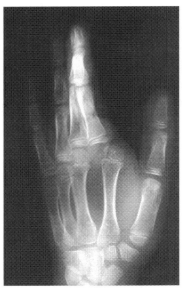

FIG 11—Oblique view of the hand showing a dislocation of the index finger metacarpophalangeal joint.

The hand

The standard radiographic projections of the whole hand are required to evaluate the base of the proximal phalanges and the metacarpals. When the injury is confined to the distal end of a single digit radiography should be limited to that digit, but the same projections are used.

Posteroanterior view should show the whole of the hand including the base of the metacarpals. It forms the basis of all assessments but is poor at showing fractures of the articular surface of the metacarpal head.

Lateral view—In this projection the metacarpal bones and phalanges are superimposed and can obscure each other. The problem can be partially overcome by flexing the fingers like a fan. The view is essential to show displacement of fracture fragments and joint dislocations.

Posteroanterior oblique view—For complete assessment this view should be requested together with posteroanterior and lateral views. It is particularly useful for assessing dislocation of the metacarpophalangeal and carpometacarpal joints and fractures at the base of the metacarpal bones (fig 11).

The thumb

The standard views of the hand do not give true posteroanterior and lateral projections of the thumb because the plane of the thumb is at 90° to the fingers. Separate posteroanterior and lateral views of the thumb should be requested. When taken correctly they greatly improve visualisation and recognition of injury at the base of the thumb.

System of radiographic assessment

ABCs system of radiological assessment

Adequacy
Alignment
Bones
Cartilage
Soft tissues

Radiographs of the hand should be assessed by using the ABCs system. This system can be applied to all views.

Posteroanterior view
 Check the adequacy and quality of the radiograph
 Check alignment of bones—Follow the alignment of the phalanx and metacarpal of each finger and the thumb.

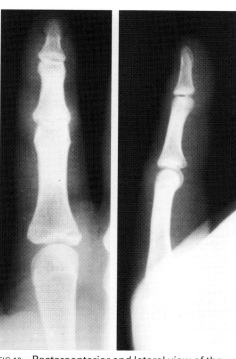

Check bone margins and density—Starting with the thumb and progressing to the fingers, metacarpals, and wrist follow the cortical margin of each bone separately in a clockwise direction. Check the bone density and trabecular pattern as you go. Vascular channels are often seen in the distal shaft of the phalanges and may be mistaken for fractures. They appear as thin, radiolucent lines that run obliquely from the external proximal surface to enter the medullary canal distally.

Check the cartilage and joints—Check each joint space in an orderly fashion, looking specifically at the congruity and separation of the margins of the joint space (fig 5). The bones should not overlap and the joint space should be uniform in width (about 1 mm). Compare injured and non-injured joints.

FIG 12—Posteroanterior and lateral view of the index finger. The fracture of the base of the proximal phalanx is visible only in the posteroanterior view. The lateral view is inadequate as it does not show the metacarpophalangeal joint.

Catches to avoid

If not true the posteroanterior view may:
• Miss an avulsion fracture affecting the collateral ligament
• Cause soft tissue shadows of the web space to look like a fracture line. The line extends past the cortical margin of the bone and beyond into the soft tissues

If not true the lateral view may miss:
• A joint dislocation
• Avulsion fracture of volar plate
• Fracture through the articular surface of the base of a phalanx

Check the soft tissues—Soft tissue abnormalities are best seen by using a bright light. Although foreign bodies may be seen in this view, tangential views will remove the superimposed bone shadow and increase the likelihood of visualisation. Soft tissue swelling may be the only indicator of injury.

Summary
History including detailed mechanism of injury
Meticulous clinical examination
Appropriate radiograph and systematic assessment with ABCs system

WRIST

D W Hodgkinson, N Kurdy, D A Nicholson, P A Driscoll

> Most injuries to the wrist result from a fall on an outstretched hand

The wrist is composed of eight bones arranged in a proximal row (scaphoid, lunate, triquetrum, and pisiform) and distal row (trapezium, trapezoid, capitate, and hamate). Each row functions as a separate unit. Three articulations make up the carpus (figs 1 and 2).

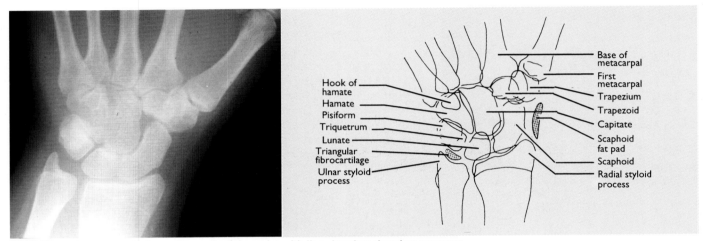

FIG 1—Normal posteroanterior radiograph of the wrist with line drawing showing anatomy.

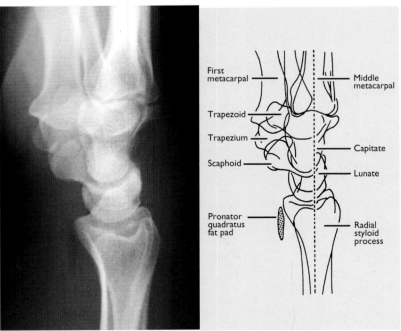

FIG 2—Normal lateral radiograph of the wrist with line drawing showing anatomy.

Radiocarpal joint—The distal radius articulates with the bones of the proximal carpal row (except the pisiform and triquetrum). This joint complex is supported by strong radiocarpal and intercarpal ligaments.

Carpocarpal joints—The proximal carpal row articulates with the distal row. These articulations are also supported by strong intercarpal ligaments that can be damaged in isolation after wrist sprains or in combination with scaphoid fractures and carpal dislocations.

Carpometacarpal joints—The distal carpal row articulates with the proximal end of the metacarpal bones. The finger carpometacarpal joints allow little movement compared with that of the thumb.

The carpal bones are bound to each other by short intercarpal ligaments, such as the scapholunate and the triquetrolunate. The articulation of the distal radioulnar joint including the triangular fibrocartilage allows pronation and supination at the wrist joint.

Foreign bodies such as wood are often
non-radio-opaque and therefore are not
visible on standard radiography

Development

Primary ossification centres of the carpus begin to appear at 3
months of age, starting with the capitate and hamate. By the age of 5-6
years all the carpal bones have visible ossification centres. The last
bones to ossify are the scaphoid and trapezoid.

Mechanisms of common injury

Most injuries to the wrist are caused by a fall on the outstretched
hand. This results in dorsiflexion and ulnar deviation of the hand
together with supination of the carpus against a pronated forearm. The
resultant force is focused across the waist of the scaphoid and the
carpocarpal joint. The injury depends on the age of the patient, the
severity and type of force, and the point of impact.

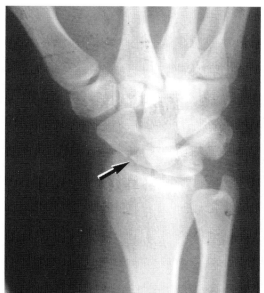

FIG 3—Oblique view of wrist showing a fracture
through the waist of the scaphoid (arrow).

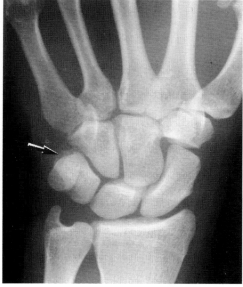

FIG 4—Posteroanterior view
showing a fracture of the
triquetrum (arrow).

Carpal fractures

Wrist fractures usually occur in people aged 15-40 years. The
scaphoid is the most commonly fractured carpal bone (fig 3). Good
quality scaphoid views will allow most scaphoid fractures to be
identified from the initial films. If clinical suspicion remains, more
specific imaging may be necessary. The triquetrum is the second
commonest carpal bone to be fractured (fig 4).

Carpal dislocations

These are uncommon injuries but may be associated with a carpal
fracture. The commonest carpal dislocations are the lunate, the lunate
with a scaphoid fracture, and the perilunate (fig 5). The relation of the
lunate to the distal radius is best seen in the lateral view (fig 6).

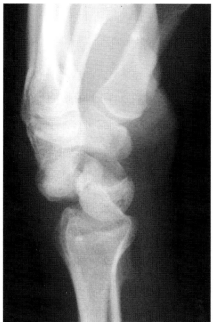

FIG 5—Lateral view of the wrist showing
a perilunate dislocation.

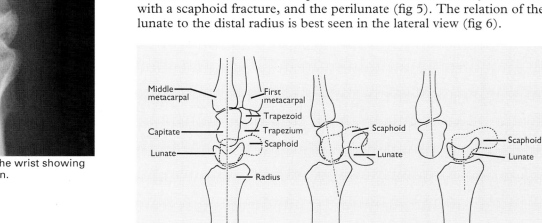

FIG 6—Dislocations of the wrist. Left, normal lateral anatomy; middle, lunate
dislocation; right, perilunate dislocation.

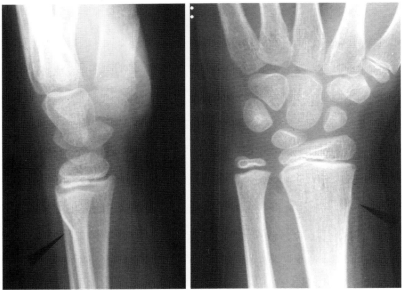

FIG 7—Lateral and posteroanterior of the wrist showing a torus fracture of the distal radial metaphysis (arrows).

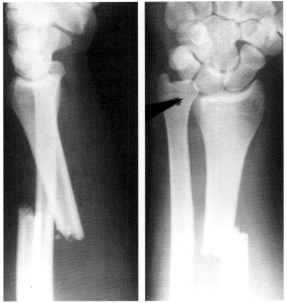

FIG 8—Lateral and posteroanterior wrist views showing Glaeazzi's fracture dislocation. This is a fracture of the shaft of the radius with disruption of the distal radial-ulnar joint (arrow).

Fractures of the distal radius and ulna

Colles' fractures are common in middle aged and elderly women. Always look for other associated injuries such as concomitant scaphoid fractures. Epiphyseal and distal metaphyseal injuries are common in children. In most cases the fracture is evident. In children minimal greenstick fractures and epiphyseal injuries can be difficult to identify (look at the cortical margin, trabecular pattern, and soft tissue indicators of injury).

The torus fracture refers to the appearance of a buckled cortex (fig 7). This usually occurs 2-4 cm proximal to the distal growth plate in children aged 4-10 years. It may be visible only in the lateral view on the dorsal surface of the cortex. Occasionally it can be seen in the posteroanterior view as a slight bump on the medial and lateral cortical margins.

Other important fractures in this region include Smith's fracture (which is opposite to a Colles' fracture and is differentiated from it in the lateral view) and Barton's fracture (a fracture-dislocation of the radiocarpal joint). An isolated fracture of the ulnar styloid process is rare. It usually occurs in association with the more common distal radial fractures. Isolated dislocation of the distal radioulnar joint is also uncommon but usually occurs in association with fracture of the radius (Galeazzi's fracture, fig 8). It is recognised by diastasis of the radioulnar joint, which produces apparent shortening or overriding of the distal radial articular surface in relation to the distal ulna.

Radiographic views

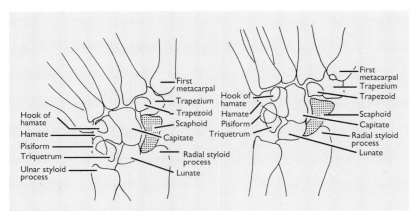

FIG 9—Line drawings showing the visibility of the carpal scaphoid on posteroanterior and anteroposterior oblique views.

Posteroanterior film—This includes the base of the metacarpals, the carpometacarpal joints, the carpocarpal joints, the radiocarpal joint, and the distal radius and ulna in profile.

The lateral view is essential for identifying dislocations of the carpus and common avulsion fractures of the dorsal surface of the triquetrum.

Posteroanterior oblique view—As well as the above projections the specific views for assessing the carpal scaphoid include the posteroanterior oblique and anteroposterior oblique, both taken with the wrist in ulnar deviation. These views maximise the visibility of the scaphoid bone and all four views are required for proper assessment (fig 9).

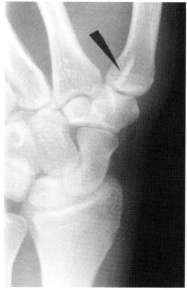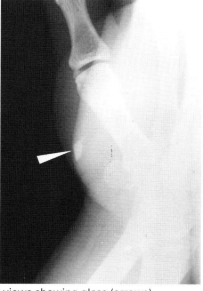

Tangential views may be used to detect foreign bodies (fig 10). More specific views of the wrist are available to suit particular problems but these would be requested only by a specialist.

FIG 10—Posteroanterior and tangential views showing glass (arrows).

System of radiographic assessment

ABCs system of radiographic assessment

Adequacy
Alignment
Bone
Cartilage and joints
Soft tissues

Check the adequacy and quality of the radiograph

Posteroanterior—Check for any rotation. There should be no overlap between the distal radius and ulnar bones. The trabeculae within the carpal bones should be visible and the bone margins should be clear and sharp. This is particularly important when assessing the carpal scaphoid, when subtle radiological signs may be obscured in poor quality films.

Lateral—Check for any rotation: the distal radius and ulna should be superimposed on each other, as should the bases of the metacarpal bones.

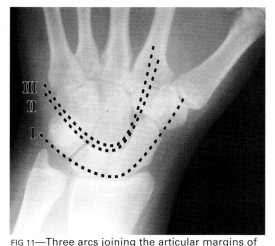

FIG 11—Three arcs joining the articular margins of the carpal bones.

Check alignment of bones

Posteroanterior—The joint margins should be parallel and the width of the joints and distance between apposing carpal bones should be 1-2 mm. Excessive widening or narrowing indicates displacement of at least one of the adjacent carpal bones. In your mind draw three parallel arcs joining the articular margins of the carpal bones (fig 11). The first arc is formed by the proximal articular margins of the proximal carpal row (the scaphoid, lunate, and triquetrum), the second by connecting the distal articular margins of the proximal carpal row, and the third by joining the proximal articular margins of the capitate and hamate. Any disruption of these parallel lines indicates subluxation or dislocation of the carpal bone. The pisiform is normally superimposed on the triquetrum.

Tracing the outline of each bone can be difficult in the lateral view because many of them are superimposed

Lateral—There should be 10-15° of volar angulation of the radiocarpal joint. The most important line to follow bisects the metacarpal base, the capitate, the lunate, and the distal radius (fig 6). The proximal pole of the capitate is inset within the lunate, and the lunate in turn is inset within the radius. Look for evidence of carpal dislocation, which will disrupt this alignment. Also assess the alignment of the thumb metacarpal to the trapezium.

Wrist

Scaphoid fat pad sign

The scaphoid fat pad sign is positive if the fat is displaced laterally away from the concave surface of the scaphoid forming a linear or convex line

---

Swelling of the soft tissue may be the only radiological indication of an injury to the wrist

---

Summary

History including detailed mechanism of injury

Meticulous clinical examination

Appropriate radiograph and systematic assessment

Check bone margins and density

Posteroanterior—Check the margins and internal trabecular pattern of each bone systematically. Start with the base of the metacarpals and work through the distal carpal row, proximal carpal row, and finally the distal radius and ulna. Look for evidence of disruption. In children the cortical margin may be only minimally disrupted, but disruption of the internal trabecular pattern may be more pronounced. When looking for a carpal scaphoid fracture check the bone margin of the articular cortex opposite the capitate. If there is no disruption, a fracture is unlikely.

Lateral—This is the best view to detect carpal and metacarpal dislocations and fracture of the triquetrum and distal radius. Avulsion of a bone fragment from the site of insertion of the dorsal radiocarpal ligament into the triquetrum often occurs after flexion at the wrist.

Check the cartilage and joints

Posteroanterior—Check the distal radioulnar joint for evidence of diastasis as in Galeazzi's fracture. Then check the orientation and relationship of each of the carpal bones. Take particular note of the scapholunate joint. An increase in the joint space may indicate carpal instability or perilunate or lunate dislocation, or both.

Lateral—Look at the orientation of the lunate (fig 5).

Check the soft tissues

Posteroanterior—A bright light is needed to see soft tissue swelling. The scaphoid fat pad is a linear collection of fat located between the radial collateral ligament and the synovial tendon sheaths of the extensor pollicis brevis and the abductor pollicis longus. It is not seen consistently in children under 12 years old. A positive scaphoid fat pad sign is a useful indicator of injury on the radial side of the wrist. It should not be used alone to confirm the presence or absence of a scaphoid fracture. Check for foreign bodies. Tangential views may help visualisation by removing superimposed bone shadows (fig 10).

Lateral—An abnormal pronator quadratus shadow on the volar aspect of the wrist (anterior bowing >1 cm from the volar cortical margin of the distal radius or obliterated) may be the only radiological sign of a distal forearm injury in children and adults (fig 2). This shadow is visible because of a thin layer of adipose tissue overlying the muscle belly.

ELBOW

D A Nicholson, P A Driscoll

The elbow is a commonly injured joint in both children and adults. Interpretation of elbow radiographs is sometimes difficult because of the complex anatomy and obscurity of certain injuries. Errors can be avoided by using a systematic approach to interpreting radiographs based on knowledge of the important anatomical relations.

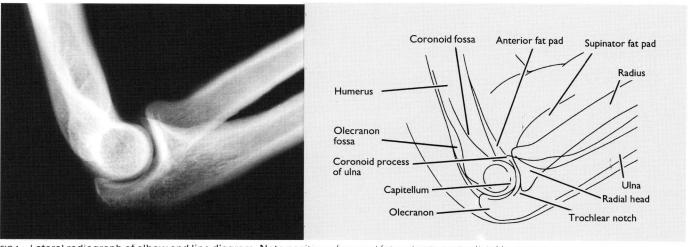

FIG 1—Lateral radiograph of elbow and line diagram. Note position of normal fat pad anterior to distal humerus.

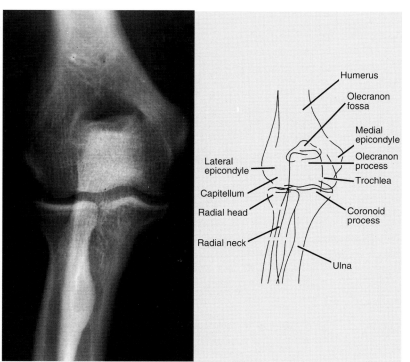

FIG 2—Anteroposterior radiograph of right elbow and line diagram.

Adult

The elbow is composed of three joints: the humeroulnar, humeroradial, and radioulnar. All are contained in a single synovial cavity. The lower end of the humerus consists of a spherical portion (capitellum), which articulates with the radius, and a grooved portion (trochlea), which articulates with the ulna. The capitellum and trochlear portions of the humerus are at about 45° to the shaft, so that a line projected along the anterior humeral cortex should intersect the middle of the ossification centre of the capitellum (fig 4).

The elbow ligaments consist of the ulnar collateral (medial), radial collateral (lateral), and annular ligaments. The annular ligament is attached to the ulna and clasps the head and neck of the radius in the superior radioulnar joint. There is no attachment to the radius, which is free to rotate in the annular ligament (fig 3).

11

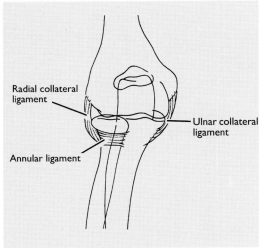

FIG 3—Ligaments of the elbow.

The capsule is attached to the humerus at the margins of the articular surfaces of the capitellum and trochlea. In front and behind it is carried above the coronoid and olecranon fossae. Distally the capsule is attached to the trochlear notch of the ulna and to the annular ligament, with no attachment to the radius. The capsule comprises an inner synovium and an outer fibrous layer separated by a layer of fat; this forms the basis of the "fat pad signs." Normally, only the anterior distal humeral fat is visible as the posterior fat is depressed within the olecranon fossa (fig 1). The supinator fat plane is identified as a radiolucent line parallel to the cortex of the proximal third of the radius. In most adults it is within 1 cm of the cortex of the radius (fig 1).

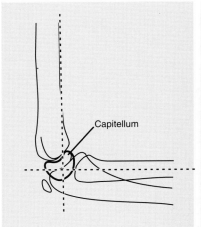

FIG 4—Line diagram showing anterior humeral line and central radial lines. These are two important lines which identify normal anatomical relations and are valuable in assessing fractures and dislocation. Both these lines intersect the middle third of the capitellum.

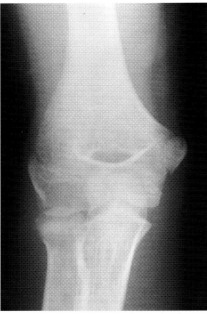

FIG 5—Anteroposterior radiograph of 12 year old child showing secondary growth centres.

Children

Epiphysial growth in the elbow is complex. The first secondary growth centre to appear in the humerus is the capitellum at about 2 years (fig 4). The medial epicondyle is the next humeral centre to appear (age 4-7 years) and is seen well before ossification of the lateral epicondyle (fig 5). The accessory ossification apophysis of the olecranon appears between the ages of 8 and 11 and usually fuses by the age of 14.

Mechanism of common types of injury

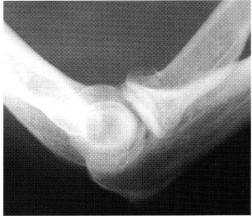

FIG 6—Anterior positive fat pad sign in a patient with a radial neck fracture—a subtle break is seen through the radial neck with disruption of the normal smooth cortical curve.

Most elbow injuries are caused by indirect trauma transmitted through the bones of the forearm. Direct blows account for very few fractures or dislocations.

Soft tissues

Soft tissue changes are often the most obvious radiological abnormality after trauma to the elbow. A positive fat pad sign is always seen with intracapsular injuries of the elbow as intra-articular haemorrhage causes distension of the synovium and displacement of the fat (fig 6). However, in severe injuries the anterior fat pad may be obliterated because of associated haemorrhage and oedema of the capsule.

Pulled elbow

Pulled elbow is common between the ages of 2 and 4 years, occurring when the child is lifted by the hand or wrist. It is due to subluxation of the radial head out of the annular ligament. Subluxation is diagnosed on clinical findings as the radial epiphysis is not ossified at this age.

Supracondylar fracture

This is the most common fracture in children, accounting for 60% of childhood fractures. It is usually caused by a fall on the outstretched hand. In most cases the transverse fracture line is easily identified but the distal epiphysis can cause confusion in some cases. There is usually posterior displacement of the distal fragment with the anterior humeral line passing through the anterior third of the capitellum or entirely anterior to it. However, a quarter of incomplete fractures show little displacement and may be overlooked.

Causes of fat pad sign

Haemorrhage

Inflammation

Trauma—found in over 90% of intra-articular skeletal injuries

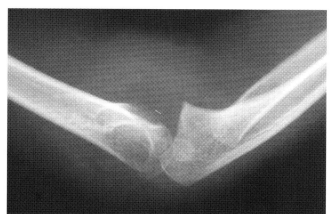

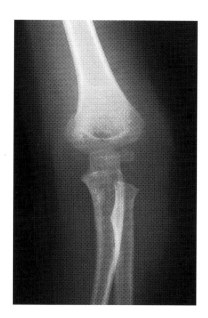

FIG 7—Left: Lateral radiograph showing a supracondylar fracture in the left elbow of a child. There is a large joint effusion with positive anterior and posterior fat pad signs. Minimal cortical disruption is seen on the posterior aspect of the lower humerus but there is posterior displacement of the distal fragment with the anterior humeral line passing anterior to the capitellum. Right: Anteroposterior radiograph of the elbow shows a subtle break in the medial cortex representing the supracondylar fracture.

This fracture is always associated with a positive fat pad sign unless the joint capsule is severely disrupted or torn. In about 5% of supracondylar fractures (usually greenstick) the anterior humeral line is normal. Look for subtle buckling of the cortex (fig 7). Occasionally oblique views may be needed to confirm the fracture line.

Epicondylar injuries

Fracture of the lateral humeral epicondyle is the second most common fracture in children, occurring in 15% (fig 8).

Half of avulsions of the medial epicondylar apophysis are associated with dislocation of the elbow. Avulsion can occur as an isolated injury due to a valgus stress during a fall on the outstretched hand or, less commonly, to repeated moderate contractions or a single violent contraction of the flexure muscles of the forearm.

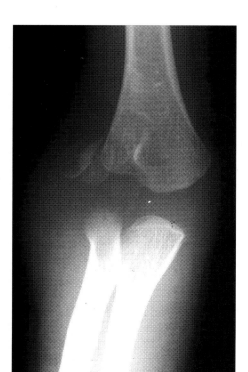

FIG 8—Fracture and dislocation of lateral humeral epicondyl and capitellum. Note the severe swelling of soft tissue.

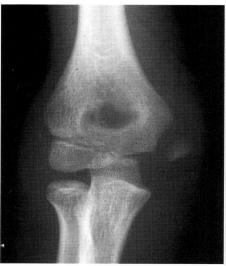
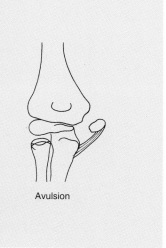

Avulsion

FIG 9—Left: Anteroposterior radiograph and line diagram of right elbow avulsion of medial epicondyle with associated soft tissue swelling.

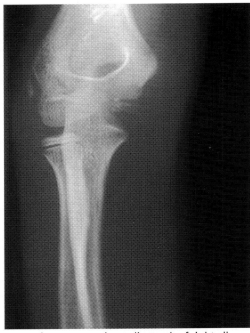

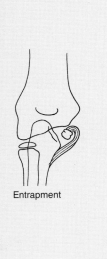

Entrapment

The avulsed medial epicondyle is almost always displaced inferiorly but some anterior or posterior displacement can also occur (fig 9). Localised soft tissue swelling is always seen. The avulsed epicondyle may be drawn into the joint space between the trochlea and the coronoid process of the ulna causing entrapment (fig 10). Such avulsion is clinically important and usually requires open reduction and internal fixation. In subtle cases a radiograph of the non-injured side may be needed for comparison. As the medial apophysis is intracapsular this separation produces a positive fat pad sign.

FIG 10—Anteroposterior radiograph of right elbow. The medial apophysis is missing and the lateral apophysis is ossified. Entrapment of the medial apophysis can be seen between the trochlea and ulna.

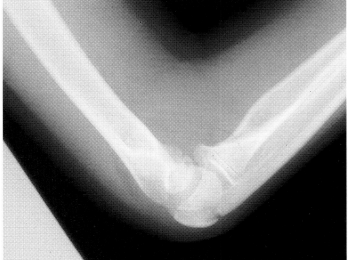

FIG 11—Slightly displaced fracture through the distal humerus of the left elbow.

Radial head or neck fractures

Fracture of the radial head is the most common injury in adults (fig 6), accounting for about half of all fractures about the elbow. Both head and neck fractures are caused by a fall on the outstretched hand with the forearm in supination. Displacement in radial neck fractures varies and they can be impacted. Often no cortical break is seen and only a slight angulation of the normally smooth concave cortex of the radial neck can be detected. It is therefore important to identify the secondary signs; virtually all radial head or neck fractures are associated with positive anterior and posterior fat pad signs and displacement or obliteration of the supinator fat plane. Radial head fractures may be classified as linear non-displaced, marginal, depressed, or comminuted.

Fractures of olecranon

Fractures of the olecranon account for a fifth of elbow injuries in adults. They occur either indirectly by a fall on the outstretched hand with the elbow flexed or directly by a blow to the olecranon. The fracture line is usually transverse passing into the trochlear notch (fig 12). Occasionally the olecranon is comminuted and distracted. Associated soft tissue swelling of the olecranon bursa is an important sign when the fracture line is undisplaced.

Fractures of long bones

Fractures of the distal humerus in adults occur after a fall on the flexed elbow. The trochlear ridge of the ulna is impacted against the trochlear groove of the humerus, causing a T or Y shaped fracture of the distal humerus. If an angular force is applied during injury an oblique epicondylar fracture may occur (fig 11). Transcondylar fractures are rare but occur in elderly people with osteoporotic bones. The fractures may be undisplaced and difficult to identify.

FIG 12—Fracture of the olecranon appears as a verticle lucent line. Note the joint effusion, which is shown by positive anterior and posterior fat pad signs.

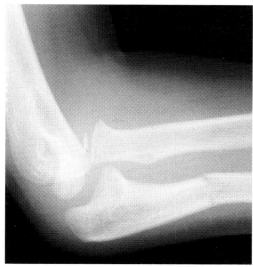

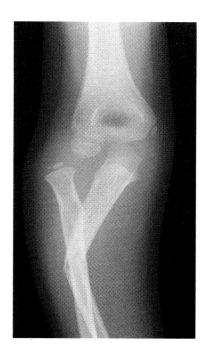

FIG 13—Lateral (left) and anteroposterior (right) radiographs of right elbow showing Monteggia's fracture. Note the obvious angulated fracture of the proximal shaft of the ulna. The central radial line passes beyond the capitellum, indicating anterior dislocation of the radius.

Monteggia's fracture

Monteggia's fracture is a fracture of the proximal third of the ulna with anterior angulation at the fracture site and anterior dislocation of the radial head (fig 13). Most result from a fall on the outstretched hand with forced pronation of the forearm, the minority occurring after a direct blow to the posterior aspect of the proximal forearm.

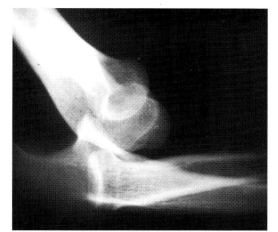

FIG 14—Posterior dislocation of elbow.

Dislocation

Backward displacement of the radius and ulna with respect to the humerus is the commonest type of dislocation, usually due to valgus angulation forces. In half of dislocations there is also a fracture of the medial epicondyle, radial head or neck, or coronoid process of the ulna. These fractures are commonly only identified in radiographs taken after reduction and are important because they represent loose bodies within the joint space that can impede complete reduction or lead to post-traumatic arthritis. Post-reduction radiographs should be taken routinely.

Types of view

Radiographic projections
Standard
Anteroposterior (fig 2)
Lateral (fig 1)
Additional
Obliques

The routine projections of the elbow include the anteroposterior and lateral. The anteroposterior view is taken with the arm fully extended and the lateral with the arm flexed to 90°. Correct positioning of the elbow is essential for interpretation as minor degrees of obliquity or rotation can obscure a positive fat pad sign or incorrectly identify the alignment of fracture fragments. Supplementary oblique views are occasionally valuable for further assessment of subtle injuries of the radial head and distal humerus.

A single projection of a long bone is inadequate to assess trauma. Films at right angles must be taken to assess displacement and decide on management. The entire long bone should be included in the film.

System of radiological assessment

ABCs system of radiological assessment

Adequacy

Alignment

Bones

Cartilage

Soft tissue

Catches to avoid

● Epiphysial lines and epiphyses can cause confusion (fig 4). Radiographs of the unaffected elbow may help

● Entrapment of the medial epicondyle can be mistaken for the ossification centre of the trochlea but this centre is irregular and never ossifies before the medial epicondyle (fig 11)

● Fracture of the lateral humeral epicondyle can be mistaken for the radiolucency of the epiphysis

● The radial tuberosity can be misinterpreted as a lucent lesion on the lateral radiograph

Summary

Check the adequacy and quality of the radiograph

Check alignment of bones
Anterior humeral line
Central radial line
Elbow joint

Check bone margins and density
Humerus
Radius
Ulna

Check the cartilage and joints

Check the soft tissues
Anterior and posterior fat pads
Supinator fat pad

Lateral radiograph

The ABCs system of radiological interpretation should be followed.

Check the adequacy and quality of the radiograph—The lateral radiograph is the most important projection as it gives most information on abnormalities of bones and soft tissues. Optimum positioning is essential so that the structures can be adequately assessed. After acute trauma, however, it can be impossible to position the patient optimally. The trochlea and capitellum should be superimposed, indicating there is no humeral rotation. When the forearm is correctly supinated the proximal shaft of the radius should be projected above the ulna. In adequately exposed radiographs the normal muscle and fascial planes are identified as linear or curvilinear radiolucent shadows because of the surrounding adipose tissue.

Check alignment of bones—Check the anterior humeral and central radial lines. The notch of the olecranon process of the ulna and the trochlea of the humerus should be in line. The coranoid process of the ulna is superimposed on the radial head.

Check bone margins and density—Examine the cortical surfaces of the humerus, radius, and ulna clockwise. Subtle breaks in children with supracondylar fractures can be difficult to detect (fig 7). Examine the internal trabecular pattern of the bones for radiolucencies or bands of increased density. Impacted radial neck fractures cause a faint broad transverse band of increased density at the junction of the head and the neck.

Check the cartilage and joints—The trochlea should be concentric to the ulna. Note the capitellum is superimposed over this joint.

Check the soft tissues—The normal anterior fat pad appears as a thin elongated radiolucency parallel and adjacent to the distal humeral cortex. A positive fat pad sign may occur when there is intra-articular fluid from any cause, including haemarthrosis after trauma. The displaced fat is seen as triangular shaped radiolucent shadows anterior and posterior to the distal end of the humerus (figs 7 and 13). A positive anterior fat pad sign indicates injury only when it is raised and becomes more perpendicular to the anterior humeral cortex. A positive posterior fat pad sign always indicates injury. Check the supinator fat plane; this may be altered or obliterated by trauma (especially radial head or neck fractures) or inflammatory processes. Check the olecranon bursa for collection of fluid.

Anteroposterior radiograph

Check alignment of bones—The relative positions of the elbow joint are easily seen in this projection.

Check bone margins and density—The cortex of the radial neck and head should form a smooth continuous concave arc extending from the radial shaft to the base of the radial head. The cortical margin of the radial head should be sharply defined. About half of radial head fractures are undisplaced, making it difficult to identify the fracture line. Subtle cortical disruptions, depressions, or steps should be carefully assessed. The articulating surface of the radius is continuous with the capitellum. Check the presence and position of the medial epicondyle. Absence of the medial epicondyle may be due to avulsion and entrapment of the centre (figs 9 and 10).

Check the cartilage and joints—The joint margin of the distal humerus appears scalloped because of the rounded capitellum and the medial and lateral borders of the trochlea. With avulsion and entrapment of the medial epicondyle there is often subtle widening of the elbow joint medially.

Check the soft tissues—Severe swelling of medial soft tissue always occurs in medial epicondylar injuries (fig 10).

SHOULDER

D A Nicholson, I Lang, P Hughes, P A Driscoll

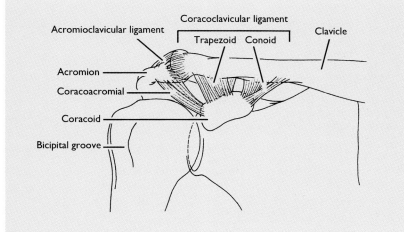

FIG 1—Diagram of shoulder ligaments.

Trauma to the shoulder is common, although the type of injury varies considerably in different age groups. Clavicular fractures are common in childhood and early adulthood, glenohumeral dislocation and acromioclavicular disruption are frequent between the ages of 15 and 40 years, and fracture of the humeral head is often seen in elderly people. This chapter describes the features of these types of injury and a system of radiological interpretation to ensure that many of the subtle signs associated with these injuries are not missed.

Important anatomical considerations

Normal measurements of acromioclavicular joint

Joint distance <8 mm
Difference between sides <3 mm

Adult

The shoulder consists of three bones and three joints. The acromion, coracoid process, and clavicle are linked by the shoulder ligaments. The coracoclavicular ligament is important as it is the main ligamentous attachment of the upper limb to the trunk. The acromioclavicular ligament is of secondary importance, but it is where radiographic evidence of injury is initially sought (fig 1).

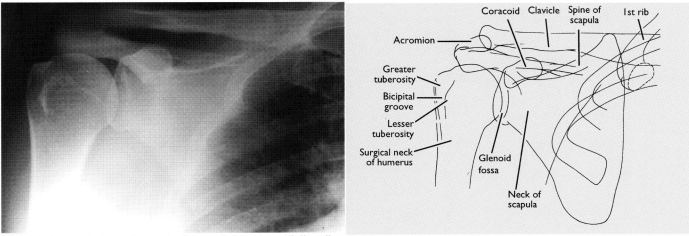

FIG 2—Anteroposterior radiograph of normal shoulder with line diagram.

Characteristics of an epiphyseal line

Dense sclerotic margins

Variable width of epiphysis

Typical anatomical location

The inferior cortex of the most lateral aspect of the clavicle usually lies in the same plane as the inferior cortex of the acromion (fig 2). The distance from the coracoid process to the undersurface of the clavicle is 11-13 mm, with a difference in sides greater than 5 mm indicating rupture. The humeral head has two tuberosities and two necks; the surgical neck is the constricted portion distal to the level of the tuberosities. The neurovascular bundle (axillary artery and vein and median, ulnar, and radial nerves) lies anterior to the glenohumeral joint and can be injured in anterior dislocation of the shoulder joint or in displaced fractures of the surgical neck.

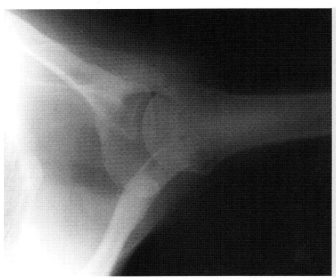
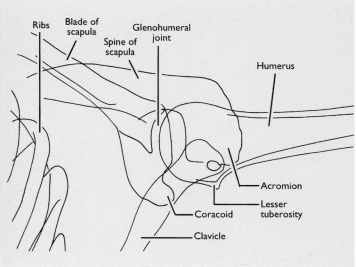

FIG 3—Axial projection of normal left shoulder with line diagram.

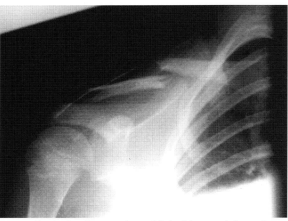

FIG 4—Clavicular fracture in a child with overriding of fracture site. Note the normal humeral epiphysis. The artefact over the shoulder is due to a dressing.

Children and development

The three epiphyseal centres of the humeral head, greater tuberosity, and lesser tuberosity fuse with one another in the sixth year and with the shaft of the humerus in the 20th year (fig 4).

The apophysis at the acromion appears at the age of 15 and is united within five years. The ossification centre at the interior angle of the scapula is generally seen between the ages of 15 and 25 years.

Common injury arising from trauma

Incidence of dislocation about the shoulder

Glenohumeral (anterior 95%, posterior 5%)	85%
Acromioclavicular	13%
Sternoclavicular	2%

Ligaments

Injury to the acromioclavicular-coracoclavicular ligament complex is classified according to the degree of disruption. Grade 1 injury is stable as the coracoclavicular ligament remains intact. As the injuring force increases, the acromioclavicular ligament is completely torn, with the coracoclavicular ligament either remaining intact or partially disrupted (grade 2). Stress views of the joint may be required to diagnose grade 1 and 2 injuries. Complete disruption of both acromioclavicular and coracoclavicular ligaments is termed grade 3 (fig 5).

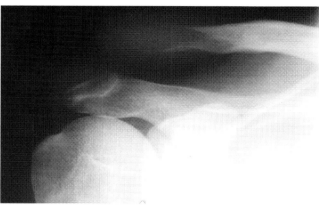

FIG 5—Disruption of acromioclavicular-coracoclavicular joint showing widening of both joints.

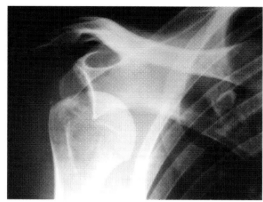

FIG 6—Anteroposterior radiograph showing anterior glenohumeral dislocation with associated chip fracture of the greater tuberosity.

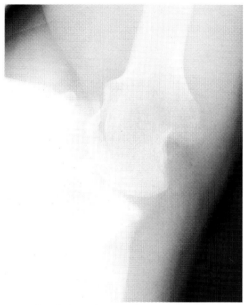

FIG 7—Axial view showing large defect in humeral head due to previous anterior dislocation and impaction fracture (Hatchet deformity).

Sternoclavicular disruption is uncommon but important because of associated vascular damage. This joint is not adequately seen in standard radiographs of the shoulder and specific views are therefore required if this injury is suspected clinically. Injury is usually suspected if chest radiography shows superior displacement of the medial end of the clavicle.

Glenohumeral dislocation

The shoulder is the most frequently dislocated joint of the body. Dislocations are usually clinically evident but radiography is needed to determine the direction of dislocation and the presence of any associated fracture or loose body (fig 6). Dislocations are classified according to the position of the humeral head with respect to the glenoid fossa.

Anterior dislocations usually occur during excessive external rotation with the arm in abduction. Occasionally the injury is due to a direct posterolateral blow. Recurrent anterior dislocation is common and is indirectly related to age (80% in people aged below 20 years and 10% in those over 40).

About 60% of patients with anterior dislocations will also have compression fractures of the upper aspect of the humeral head, resulting in a flattened segment referred to as a hatchet deformity (Hill-Sachs) (fig 7). The fracture is caused by forceful impaction of the superolateral aspect of the humerus against the anterior or inferior rim of the glenoid fossa. It is often only seen in an axial or postreduction radiograph and is best seen with internal rotation of the arm. Anterior dislocation can also be associated with fractures of the greater tuberosity of the humerus (15%) and with fractures of the anterior rim of the glenoid fossa.

Direct posterior dislocation of the shoulder is uncommon but is a major diagnostic problem. Up to half are not recognised in the initial anteroposterior film. The posterior dislocation is typically associated with an anteromedial fracture of the humeral head. Simultaneous bilateral posterior dislocations are infrequent, occurring most commonly in patients with epilepsy.

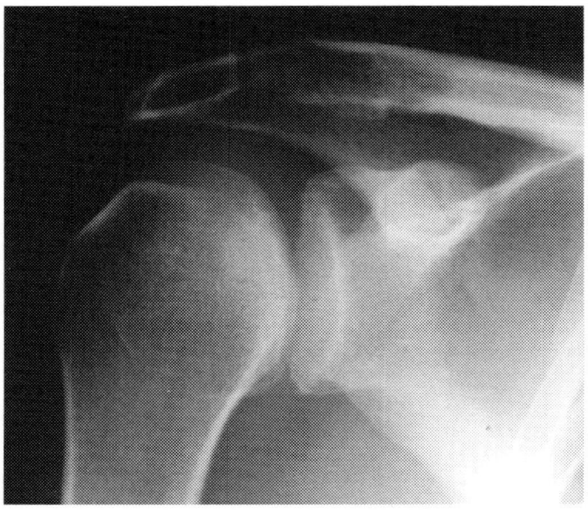

Fractures

Fractures of the shoulder can occur at the proximal humerus or glenoid fossa and may be associated with dislocation (figs 6-9). Fractures can be classified as non-displaced, displaced, or impacted. Intra-articular fractures are often associated with joint effusions or lipohaemarthrosis (fig 10).

FIG 8—Anteroposterior radiograph showing posterior glenohumeral dislocation.

Shoulder

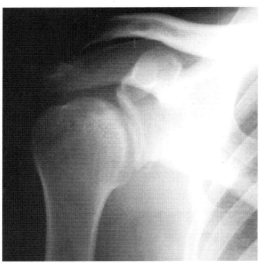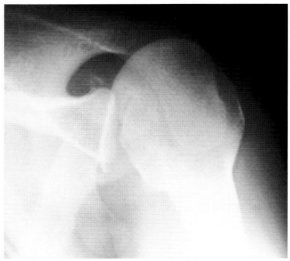

FIG 9—Left: Anteroposterior radiograph showing trough sign of posterior dislocation with associated chip fracture of the inferior glenoid fossa. Right: Axial view confirms posterior dislocation. There is a typical anteromedial fracture of the humeral head and a small fragment from the glenoid fossa.

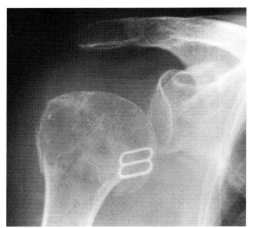

FIG 10—Fracture of humeral head showing lipohaemarthrosis. Note the humeral head is displaced inferolaterally in relation to the glenoid fossa—pseudosubluxation.

Clavicle

Clavicular fractures are common and usually follow a fall on the shoulder or outstretched hand. About 80% of fractures occur at the mid-third of the clavicle and are transverse (fig 4). Typically there is overriding of the fracture with the distal fragment being displaced inferiorly by the weight of the upper limb. Fractures of the outer third of the clavicle are also usually transverse but are non-displaced because of stabilisation from the acromioclavicular-coracoclavicular ligament complex. A raised proximal fragment suggests disruption of the coracoclavicular ligament.

Scapula

Fractures of the body of the scapula usually result from a direct crush-type injury and, with neck fractures, are the commonest injury of this bone. Fracture of the coracoid process is rare.

Non-traumatic lesions

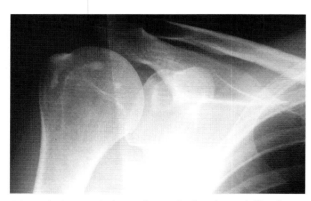

FIG 11—Anteroposterior radiograph showing calcification of the rotator cuff projected over the humerus, which appears as sclerotic areas within the humeral head. Slight calcification is seen in the soft tissues projected above the bicipital groove.

Acute or severe shoulder pain and the painful arc syndrome are often due to inflammation of a periarticular bursa or tendon. Calcification of periarticular soft tissue or of the rotator cuff muscles is often associated with this acute inflammation. Pathological fractures of the humerus through benign or malignant bone lesions may occur spontaneously or with minimal trauma.

Types of view

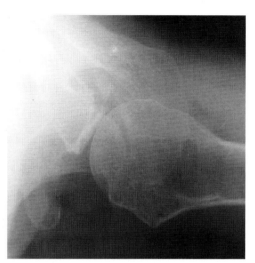

FIG 12—Axial projection showing isolated fracture of the posterior lip of the glenoid fossa. The anteroposterior projection appeared normal.

The anteroposterior radiograph is the routine view taken in all patients (fig 2). The axial projection can be modified and taken with only minimal abduction and is therefore possible in most patients, even those with severe shoulder pain.

Occasionally the radiographer is unable to position the patient for a formal axial view. In these cases a through the chest lateral view (lateral transthoracic) may be taken, although this view is most useful for assessing alignment of humeral fractures and not dislocation. The axial view provides the most information and should be taken in all patients with trauma to the shoulder (fig 12).

Stress views

When the acromioclavicular ligament is completely disrupted but the coracoclavicular ligament remains intact, separation of the bones may not occur unless the joint is stressed. If such an injury is suspected specialised stress views should be taken with the patient holding weights. The non-injured shoulder should be examined in a similar manner to act as a control.

Radiological assessment of anteroposterior radiograph

As with other radiographs the ABCs approach to interpretation is recommended.

Check the adequacy and quality of the radiograph

To take an anteroposterior shoulder view the patient is rotated slightly so that the glenohumeral joint is seen face on. The upper third of the humerus, outer half of the clavicle, and lateral aspects of the ribs should be visible.

Check alignment of bones

Firstly, check the humeral head is lying in the glenoid fossa. Then check the alignment of the acromioclavicular joint for disruption. Trace the inferior cortex of the clavicle across to the inferior cortex of the acromion. Remember partial or complete rupture of the acromioclavicular ligament can exist without disruption of the coracoclavicular ligament and can be detected only in stress views.

Check bone margins and density

Systematically trace the margins of the individual bones included in the anteroposterior projection: clavicle, humerus, scapula, and the ribs. Start at the upper aspects of each bone and work clockwise round its margin. Once you have assessed the cortex, examine the internal structure of the bones for distortion of the trabecular pattern. Difficult areas due to overlying structures include:

Humeral head—Posterior dislocation is typically associated with an anteromedial fracture of the humeral head, which is identified as a curvilinear density superimposed on the humeral head, parallel to the articulating cortex (trough sign—fig 9).

Radiological signs of posterior dislocation

1 Incongruity of the humeral head and the glenoid fossa with superimposition of the humeral head on the fossa (fig 9)
2 Positive rim sign—widening of the joint space between the head of the humerus and the anterior margin of the glenoid fossa (fig 8)
3 Light bulb sign—due to severe internal rotation of the dislocated humeral head (fig 8)
4 Trough sign—Curvilinear cortical density parallel to articulating cortex due to depressed fracture (fig 9)

The glenoid fossa, coracoid process, and body of the scapula because of overlying ribs. An avulsion fracture of the anteroinferior lip of the glenoid fossa is a common complication of dislocation of the shoulder.

Fractures of the inner third of the clavicle are uncommon and may be missed because of superimposition of the ribs.

Check cartilage and joints

The glenohumeral joint should be examined carefully as posterior dislocation of the shoulder joint may look almost normal in this view. When posterior dislocation is suspected subtle radiographic signs should be sought. Always take an axial view to exclude or confirm such a dislocation. The distance from the humeral head to the anterior margin of the glenoid fossa is usually equal from top to bottom. Asymmetry can be due to dislocation or fracture. Anterior dislocation of the humerus is the most common (fig 6). Intra-articular fractures commonly cause haemarthroses or effusions which displace the head of the humerus inferolaterally—so called pseudosubluxation (fig 10).

Acromioclavicular joint—Check the acromioclavicular joint and distance from the tip of the coracoid process to the clavicle. If there is minimal widening of the joint take stress views. When the acromioclavicular joint is completely torn (grade 2) there is usually widening of the joint as well as superior displacement of the clavicle. In grade 3 injury abnormal widening of the acromioclavicular joint and increased distance between the clavicle and coracoid process can be seen in the standard anteroposterior radiograph (fig 5).

Check soft tissues

Disruption of the acromioclavicular joint is usually associated with swelling above the joint, which can be seen with the aid of a bright light. In patients who have not experienced trauma the soft tissues should be examined for calcification, although this may overlie the bones (fig 11). Look for lipohaemarthroses or effusions around the joint capsule (fig 10).

Catches to avoid

The bicipital groove of the humeral head usually appears as a sclerotic line and should not be confused with a fracture or calcification (fig 2)

The superolateral aspect of the humeral head appears to have reduced density and may look cystic

The rhomboid fossa is a normal concavity on the inferomedial aspect of the clavicle; it is often unilateral or asymmetrical and can be mistaken for an osteolytic lesion

In children the anterior and posterior aspects of the proximal humeral epiphyseal line are at variable heights and should not be confused with fractures (fig 4). In addition the coracoid and acromion apophyses may resemble avulsion fracture fragments

Assessment of the axial radiograph

This is a notoriously difficult radiograph to interpret because of its unusual projection and overlying structures (fig 3). Nevertheless, by following an ordered system the anatomy and any abnormality can be detected.

Check the adequacy and quality of the radiograph

The coracoid process, glenoid fossa, acromion process, spine of the scapula, and lesser tuberosity of the humeral head should be identifiable.

Check alignment of bones

Identify the coracoid process anteriorly and the acromion process posteriorly. The glenoid fossa is projected between these structures. The humeral head should sit within the fossa (fig 3).

Check bone margins and density

Trace the margins of the clavicle, humerus, and scapula (spine, acromion, glenoid fossa, and coracoid process) clockwise. Fractures of the coracoid process and infraspinous processes of the scapular body are clearly seen in the axial view.

Check cartilage and joints

Examine the acromioclavicular and glenohumeral joints for separation or dislocation.

Check soft tissues

Calcification of the rotator cuff can be seen more clearly in axial views (fig 11).

Summary

Adequacy and quality of the radiograph

Alignment of bones
Glenoid fossa
Acromioclavicular joint

Bone margins and density
Clavicle
Humerus
Scapula
Ribs

Cartilage and joints
Glenohumeral joint
Acromioclavicular joint

Soft tissue
Calcification
Effusions
Lipohaemarthrosis

FOOT

D A Nicholson, D O'Keeffe, P A Driscoll

> Accurate clinical assessment of injuries to the foot will avoid unnecessary exposure to *x* rays

Radiographs of the foot and ankle are often requested together, which reflects the difficulty patients and clinicians have in separating the components of the injury. Therefore, as in other injuries of the extremities, accurate clinical assessment of the site of the acute injury is essential to avoid inappropriate films being requested. This article describes an effective system by which clinicians can request appropriate radiographs and systematically analyse them.

Important anatomical considerations

Division and joints of the foot
Hindfoot—Calcaneus and talus
Chopart's joint/midtarsal joint
Midfoot—Navicular, cuboid, cuneiforms
Metatarsotarsal joint
Forefoot—Metatarsals and phalanges

Adults

The foot can be divided into three sections (forefoot, midfoot, and hindfoot). The foot articulates with the ankle joint at the junction between the inferior surface of the talus and the superior surface of the calcaneus. This is known as the subtalar joint and inversion and eversion of the hindfoot occur here.

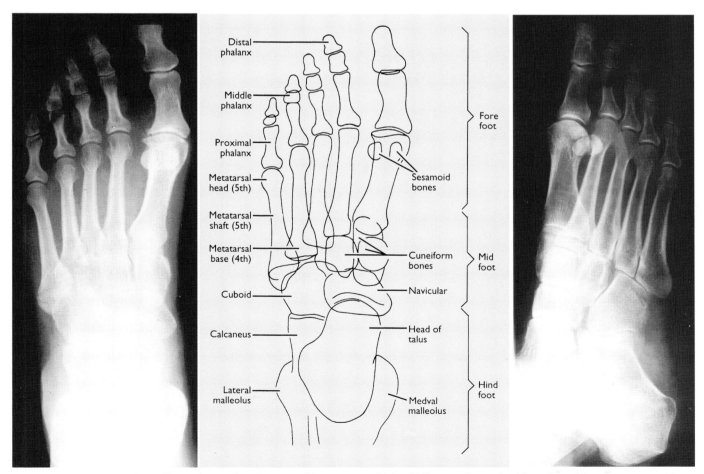

FIG 1—Left: Anteroposterior radiograph and line diagram of foot.   FIG 2—Right: Oblique radiograph of foot. Note bipartite sesamoid bone at the first metatarsophalangeal joint. There is a subtle injury (see page 27).

Foot

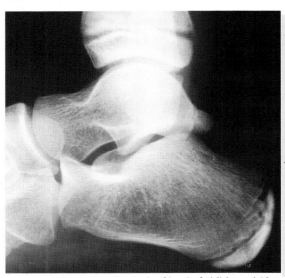

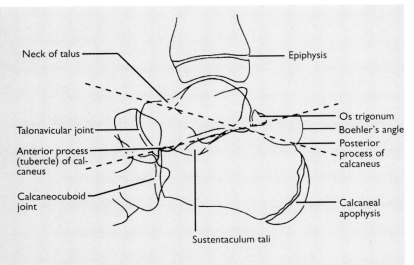

FIG 3—Left: Lateral radiograph of heel of child aged 12 years showing typical appearance of the normal calcaneal apophysis and accessory ossicle (os trigonum). The anterior and posterior calcaneal tubercles and sustentaculum tali are clear as are the subtalar, talonavicular, and calcaneocuboid joints. Right: Line diagram of radiograph showing Boehler's angle (acute angle indicated by dotted lines).

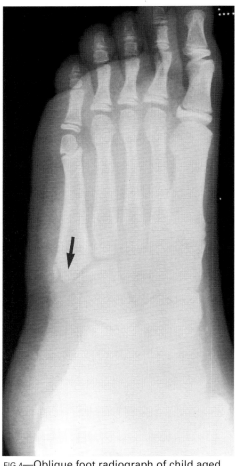

The sustentaculum tali is a large anteromedial outgrowth of the calcaneus which forms the middle articulating facet of the calcaneus and supports the head of the talus. Supination and pronation of the midfoot and forefoot takes place at the midtarsal joint. The Achilles tendon inserts into the posterior aspect of the tubercle of the calcaneus.

A clinically important structure in the metatarsotarsal joint is Lisfranc's ligament, which extends from the medial cuneiform to the base of the second metatarsal. Disruption of this ligament or fracture through the base of the metatarsals is a severe injury which causes disruption of the metatarsotarsal joint.

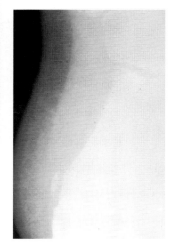

Children

The developing foot can have numerous accessory centres of ossification and named ossicles—for example, the os trigonum is present in up to 25% of normal children and is often bilateral (fig 3). Several normal variants in the foot can at first sight closely resemble fractures. A pair of sesamoid bones is normally identified on the plantar aspect of the head of the first metatarsal (figs 1 and 2). A separate ossification centre is seen arising from the medial aspect of the navicular in about 5% of children. The normal calcaneal apophysis is fragmented, irregular, and more dense than the body of the calcaneus (fig 3).

FIG 4—Oblique foot radiograph of child aged 11 years. Note the location of the epiphyses, normal fragmentation of the calcaneal apophysis (enlargement), and accessory ossification centre at the base of the fifth metatarsal along the axis of the bone. A transverse avulsion fracture is visible (arrow).

Mechanisms of common injury

Fractures of the vertebral transverse processes and wedge fractures of the upper lumbar spine are often overlooked at initial presentation in patients with calcaneal fractures caused by falling from a height

Fractures of the calcaneus are the most common tarsal fractures. They occur after compression forces and crush injuries when falling on to the feet and may be associated with contralateral fractures of the calcaneus (10%), fractures of the vertebral transverse processes, or wedge fractures of the upper lumbar spine, especially L2 (10%).

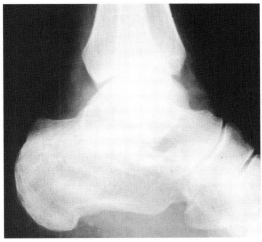

FIG 5—Lateral ankle radiograph showing linear fracture of the calcaneus, seen as a zone of radiolucency with reduction in Boehler's angle.

Thoracolumbar fractures should be considered in unconscious patients who have fallen from a height on to their feet. Many fractures of the calcaneus are obvious, but occasionally subtle fractures can be detected only by finding a reduced Boehler's angle. This is the angle subtended by the lines drawn on the lateral view of the ankle or foot from the posterior tubercle through the superior aspect of the posterior facet and a line drawn from the posterior facet to the superior margin of the anterior process (fig 3, right). Boehler's angle is normally 25-40°; an angle less than 25° indicates a depressed fracture of the subtalar portion of the calcaneus.

Seventy five per cent of calcaneal fractures affect the subtalar joints (figs 5 and 6). Fracture of the anterior process of the calcaneus is common but is often overlooked because of poor views of this region. In addition, the anterior process that arises from a secondary ossification centre may fail to unite (os secundum) and cause confusion.

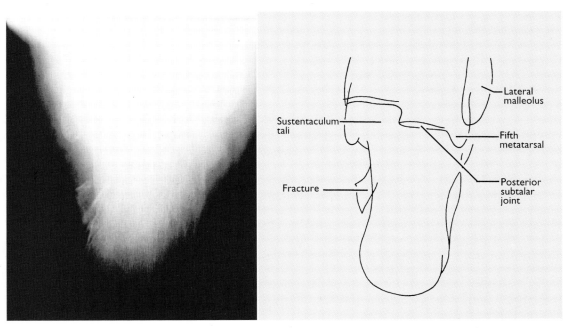

FIG 6—Axial view and line diagram of calcaneus showing displaced fracture and normal sustentaculum tali.

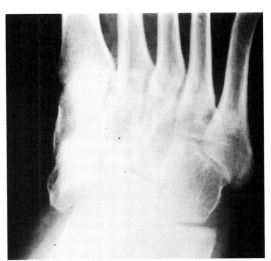

FIG 7—Fracture dislocation of the (midtarsal) talonavicular joint—Chopart's dislocation, a rare injury.

Fractures of the tarsal bones can occur after direct trauma but are uncommon. Avulsion of the dorsal or medial aspects of the navicular bone is more usual. Dislocations of the tarsus are common and are often clinically obvious; they may, however, be difficult to assess radiologically because of the complexity of the relation of the subtalar regions and tarsus (fig 7). Computed tomography is often needed to identify the displacement of the bones accurately.

Fractures and dislocations of the metatarsotarsal joint may be either homolateral or divergent (fig 8). They usually occur after massive trauma to the foot, such as in road traffic accidents or when parachute jumpers land with the foot in extended plantar flexion. In the homolateral type the lateral four metatarsals move laterally as a unit, sparing the first metatarsal. With the divergent type the first metatarsal is dislocated medially while the second to fifth metatarsals move laterally; this is occasionally associated with dislocation or fracture of the medial cuneiform. Neuropathic diabetic feet are prone to this injury.

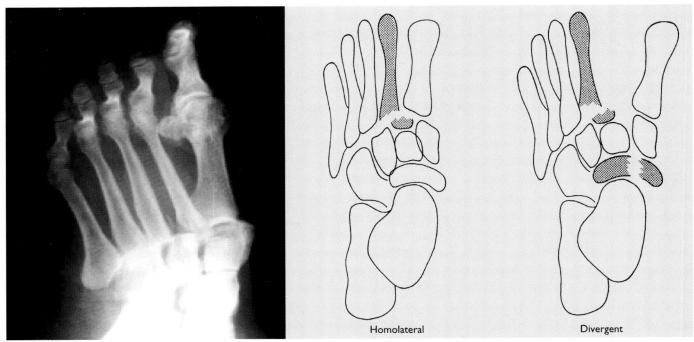

Homolateral   Divergent

FIG 8—Radiograph and line diagram showing types of injury to the metatarsotarsal joint. With the divergent type there may be associated fractures of the cuneiforms or navicular.

The area of the foot most often injured in trauma to the ankle is the base of the fifth metatarsal (figs 1 and 4). Clinically this fracture resembles a fracture of the lateral malleolus. As this part of the foot is usually included in the lateral and anteroposterior ankle views further foot radiographs are often not necessary

Fracture of the base of the fifth metatarsal results from inversion of the foot, which produces tension on the peroneus brevis attached to the base of the fifth metatarsal. This injury is sustained by stepping off a kerb or falling when walking down stairs. In most cases an avulsion fracture of the fifth metatarsal is sustained (fig 1). In some cases, however, a Jones fracture occurs. A Jones fracture affects the proximal diaphysis of the fifth metatarsal approximately 2 cm from its base. Metatarsal fractures are common and readily seen unless they are "stress fractures" (march) due to repeated subcortical trauma to a normal bone, usually the second metatarsal. Delayed films (two to three weeks after the injury) will usually show reparative periosteal new bone (fig 9). Isoptope bone scanning, however, will show a characteristic appearance after 24-48 hours.

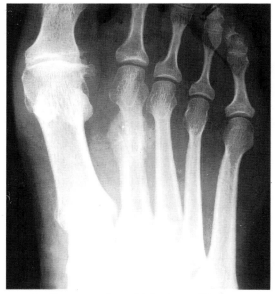

FIG 9—Healing stress (march) fracture of the second metatarsal shaft. The film at the time of onset of pain appeared normal.

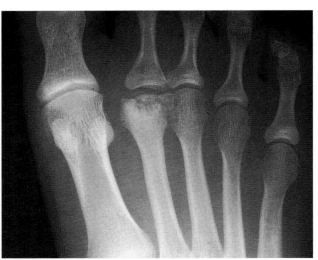

FIG 10—Freiberg's infarction of the second metatarsal head in a 14 year old girl.

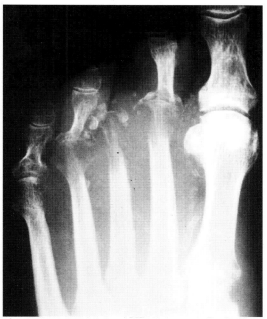

FIG 11—Severely infected diabetic foot with osteomyelitis and bony destruction of the second, third, and fourth metatarsal heads. Note vascular calcification and previous amputation of distal third toe.

Osteochondritis of the second metatarsal head (Freiberg's infarction) occurs in children (fig 10). It has a questionable relation with trauma and is detected by fragmentation of the articular surface. This heals with residual deformity but surprisingly little secondary osteoarthritis.

Osteomyelitis produces soft tissue swelling and irregular or moth eaten areas of bone destruction (fig 11). Periosteal new bone formation is also seen but it is not evident for 10-14 days; the diagnosis is therefore initially a clinical one. Specialist advice should be sought early if this condition is suspected.

Radiological assessment of the foot

Standard radiographic views

Foot:
 Anteroposterior (fig 1)
 Oblique (fig 2)

Heel (hindfoot):
 Lateral (fig 3)
 Axial (fig 6)

Catches to avoid

● Accessory ossification centres, particularly at the base of the fifth metatarsal, may cause confusion, but the accessory ossification centre runs parallel to the long axis of the foot whereas most fractures are horizontal (fig 4)

● Accessory ossification centres are usually bilateral and have smooth rounded contours with intact cortical margins c Sesamoid bones of the great toe arise from two or more centres that fail to unite and may resemble an epiphyseal fracture (fig 2)

● Radiolucencies caused by soft tissues may be seen overlying the distal foot, simulating fractures. These lines, however, extend beyond the cortical margins of the bones and are only seen in one projection (fig 12)

● The appearance of the calcaneal apophysis is extremely variable; it may look fragmented and show irregular calcification (fig 3)

● A cyst in the calcaneus caused by overlapping normal trabecular arches is normal and sh ould not be misinterpreted as indicating disease

---

Because the foot is complex both anteroposterior and oblique views are required. The lateral view has limited value because the bones appear superimposed. Axial and true lateral views of the calcaneus are taken if clinical evidence suggests it is fractured. Fractures of the subtalar region may require additional oblique views, but these should not be taken routinely.

Anteroposterior and oblique projections

Check the adequacy and quality of the radiograph—Normally the lateral cuneiform and cuboid bones are superimposed in the anteroposterior view. The lateral four metatarsals also overlap because of the normal transverse arch of the midfoot. An internally rotated oblique projection is best for showing most bones of the foot (fig 2). The metatarsophalangeal joints should be clear.

Check alignment of bones—The heads of the calcaneus and talus articulate with the cuboid and navicular respectively. The bases of the first, second, and third metatarsals align with the three cuneiform bones. The fourth and fifth metatarsal heads articulate with the cuboid. The line of the phalanges and metatarsals of each toe is straight. Malalignment of these structures adversely affects weight bearing. Complex fractures and dislocations in the tarsometatarsal area may look almost normal in some views (fig 7).

Check bone margins and density—Starting with the hindfoot trace the bone margins in a clockwise direction. The margins of both talus and calcaneus are normally partly obscured in the middle of the subtalar joint. Next look at the internal (medullary) bone structure and density. The trabeculae in the medullary canal should be uniform or change gradually. The anterior process of the calcaneus should be routinely assessed on the oblique projection to identify avulsion fractures. Follow the same technique for the midfoot and the forefoot bones. Check the base of the fifth metatarsal for a subtle avulsion fracture (see fig 1).

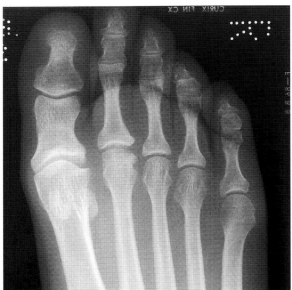

FIG 12—Fracture of fifth proximal phalanx. Note the artefacts in the overlying soft tissue which simulate fractures.

Isolated fractures of the tarsal bones other than the calcaneus are uncommon and are often obscured by the superimposition of bones. Look for subtle changes such as buckling of the cortex or a zone of increased density caused by impaction (fig 2 shows a characteristic, subtle fracture of the cuboid). The oblique view shows such fractures most clearly.

Check the cartilage and joints—Loss of joint space and increased density of superimposed bones is seen in dislocations of the subtalar, midtarsal, and metatarsotarsal joints (fig 8). Dislocation at the interphalangeal joints is usually dorsal, whereas metatarsotarsal dislocation is usually lateral or medial, causing abnormal widening at the bases of the first and second metatarsals.

Check soft tissues—Extensive soft tissue injury often accompanies severely comminuted, displaced fractures of the foot and bone infection.

Most crush calcaneal injuries cause depression of the posterior facet of the calcaneus, which reduces Boehler's angle. The angle is best assessed in a lateral radiograph of the ankle or foot

Summary

Adequacy and quality

Alignment of bones

Bone margins and density

Fractures
Boehler's angle

Cartilage and joints
Subtalar
Midtarsal
Metatarsotarsal

Soft tissues

Lateral foot projection (for examining the calcaneus)

Check the adequacy and quality of the radiograph—This view should include the ankle and midtarsal joints and is generally taken as part of the ankle series. The soft tissue overlying the calcaneus should be visible.

Check alignment of bones—Examine the talonavicular and calcaneocuboid alignment.

Check bone margins and density—Look for cortical breaks or disruption of the bony trabeculae. Curvilinear radiodense areas within the calcaneus or talus indicate overlap of cortical fragments and often are the only evidence of fracture (fig 5).

Check the cartilage and joints—Check the subtalar joint and measure Boehler's angle.

Check soft tissues—Soft tissue swelling of the heel pad can be a useful indicator of otherwise obscure fractures of the calcaneus.

ANKLE

D O'Keeffe, D A Nicholson, P A Driscoll, D Marsh

A large proportion of the radiographs performed in accident and emergency departments are for injuries to the ankle. This article describes aneffective system by which non-specialists can request appropriate radiographs and interpret them. It is essential to be familiar with the anatomy of the ankle (figs 1 and 2) and understand how it can be damaged.

> Two views of the ankle are required for proper assessment

Important anatomical considerations

Adult

The talus is the key to understanding the ankle. This bone is surrounded by a circle made of bones and ligaments. Superiorly the distal tibia is joined to the distal fibula by three ligaments (fig 3). These are the posterior and anterior tibiofibular ligaments and the interosseous membrane.

There are two important collateral ligament complexes. The collateral ligamental complexes and malleoli combine with the distal tibial articular surface to lock the talus in a mortice. Plantar flexion and dorsiflexion of the ankle occur at this joint.

> **Ankle movements**
> - Dorsiflexion and plantar flexion occur at the ankle joint
> - Inversion and eversion occur at the subtalar joint

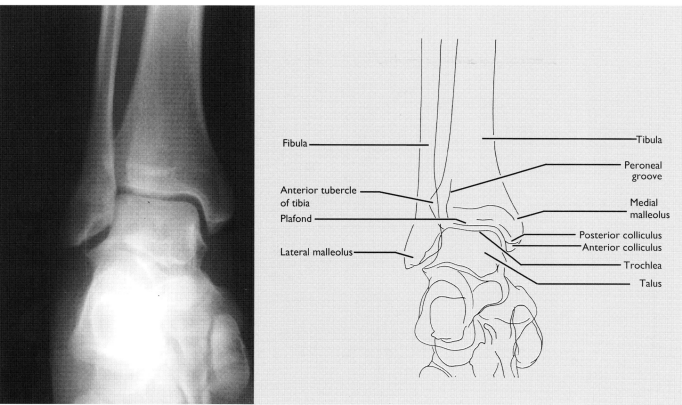

FIG 1—Normal anteroposterior ankle radiograph and line diagram.

Fibula

Anterior tubercle of tibia

Plafond

Lateral malleolus

Tibia

Peroneal groove

Medial malleolus

Posterior colliculus
Anterior colliculus

Trochlea

Talus

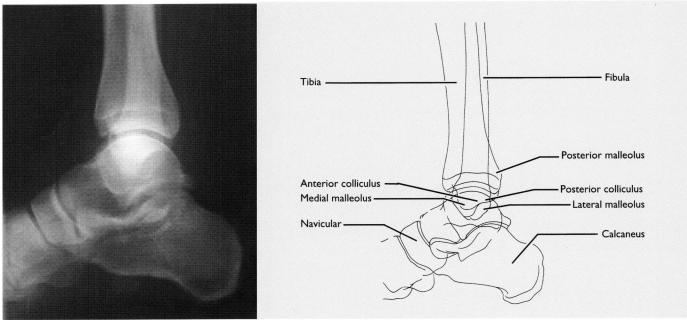

FIG 2—Normal lateral ankle radiograph and line diagram.

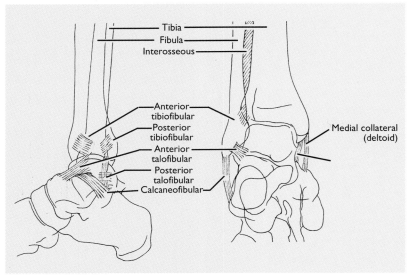

FIG 3—Line diagram of important ligaments in ankle.

The talus is divided into a body (including the dome), neck, and head. The dome has a wide anterior aspect giving it a trapezoid shape. In extreme dorsiflexion the talus is wedged between the malleoli and all the associated ligaments are taut. Therefore in this position there is little movement of the ankle mortice. This is an important factor in various types of injuries.

The talus has a vulnerable blood supply similar to the scaphoid in the wrist. As the talus has no muscular or tendinous attachments it relies on the integrity of the capsule for nutrition. The proximal part (body) receives its vascular supply from the distal aspect (head). Therefore a fracture of the waist can compromise the supply to the body, causing necrosis. Congruity of the articular surfaces is critical to the function of the joint. A 1 mm discrepancy in alignment due to a fracture leads to a 47% reduction in load bearing surfaces with consequent predisposition to degenerative joint disease.

Children

The developing ankle can have numerous accessory centres of ossification and named ossicles—for example, the os trigonum, which is present in about a quarter of the population. There is also a wide variety of normal variants that at first sight resemble fractures. Separate ossification centres have a characteristic appearance but comparison views of the other ankle are sometimes required.

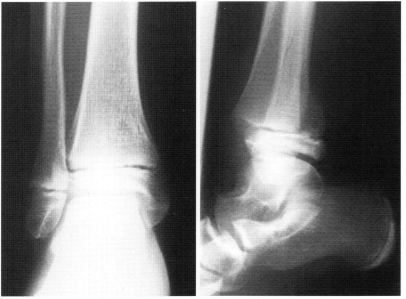

FIG 4—Anteroposterior and lateral views of child's ankle showing the importance of the two views. The anteroposterior view looks normal (note normal appearances to the epiphyses) but the lateral view shows a fracture of the posterior malleolus with posterior displacement of the epiphysis and a spiral fracture through the fibula.

Injury to a developing physis may result in premature closure of all or part of the physis with consequent deformity. Children often break the physis whereas adults strain ligaments before they break bones or dislocate joints. In children injury to a growth plate (Salter-Harris classification) requires orthopaedic attention sooner rather than later (fig 4).

> The stability of the ankle should always be investigated as this determines future management. Stability should be assessed from the mechanism of injury and the radiological findings

Stability of the ankle

Stability is lost if the circle of bones and ligaments that makes up the ankle mortice is disrupted in two or more places. Often one of the breaks will be in the supporting soft tissue and therefore not radiologically visible.

Mechanism of injury

> **Movements of the talus leading to ankle injury**
> - Movement in the coronal plane—abduction or adduction
> - Rotation about the long axis of the tibia—internal or external rotation
> - Vertical compression

Twisting ankle injuries

The ankle is almost always damaged because of abnormal movement of the talus. Occasionally only one type of movement occurs. Usually, however, a combination of these movements coexists at the time of injury. This gives rise to complex patterns of skeletal and ligamentous damage. Three patterns are distinguished according to the level and type of fibular fracture.

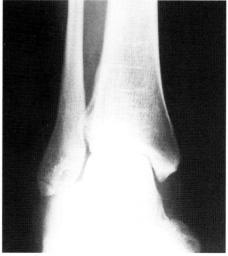

Horizontal fracture at the ankle joint or distal to it—This occurs when the main movement of the talus is adduction in the coronal plane (inversion). It leads to either tearing of the lateral collateral ligament or a horizontal avulsion fracture of the lateral malleolus (fig 5). In extreme cases the medial malleolus can be obliquely fractured (fig 6). The junction between the malleolus and the horizontal articular surface of the tibia may also be compressed. The tibiofibular ligaments remain intact and there is no diastasis of the tibiofibular joint. Avulsion most commonly occurs at the site of insertion of the anterior ankle joint capsule.

FIG 5—Radiograph showing avulsion fracture of tip of fibula.

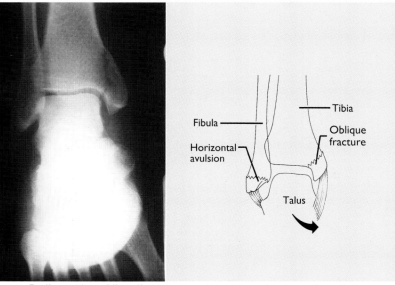

FIG 6—Radiograph and line diagram showing oblique fracture of medial malleolus with an inversion injury.

Spiral fracture at the distal tibiofibular joint or distal to it—This occurs when the main movement of the talus is abduction in the coronal plane (eversion) and rotation. It leads to a spiral fracture of the lateral malleolus, usually beginning at the ankle joint. With greater degrees of force this fracture is comminuted. The stresses in the medial collateral ligament cause it to rupture or produce a horizontal avulsion fracture of the medial malleolus (fig 7). If the talar movement continues both tibiofibular ligaments are stretched. With sufficient force the insertion of the posterior ligament into the posterior malleolus (posterior aspect of tibia) can be avulsed. The tibiofibular ligaments remain intact if the fibular fracture begins below the ankle joint.

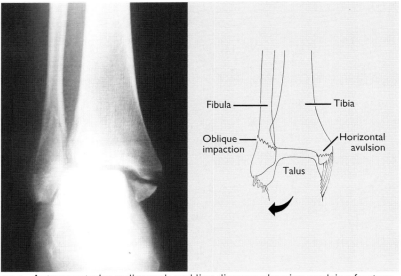

FIG 7—Anteroposterior radiograph and line diagram showing avulsion fracture of the medial malleolus and oblique fracture of the fibula. Note the lateral shift of the talus and incongruity at the ankle joint.

Fracture between the inferior tibiofibular joint and head of the fibula—This results from a combination of talar movements, the main one being external rotation. The fibula can fracture anywhere along its length—even at its neck (fig 8). Rarely the bone is preserved at the expense of dislocation of the superior tibiofibular joint. The stresses in the medial collateral ligament cause it to tear or produce a horizontal avulsion fracture of the medial malleolus. Stretching of the tibiofibular ligaments usually results in an avulsion of the posterior malleolus. The tibiofibular ligaments are torn or avulsed from their bony attachments.

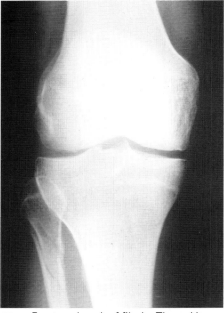

FIG 8—Fractured neck of fibula. The ankle was also fractured.

Deceleration ankle injuries

Rapid deceleration from a fall or road traffic accident can produce a force which dorsiflexes the ankle. The wide anterior aspect of the talus is driven between the malleoli, fracturing the medial one. With further dorsiflexion the anterior surface of the tibia is broken along with the lateral malleolus. If the foot is plantar flexed at the time of impact the talus strikes the posterior articular surface of the tibia, which can fracture. The fragment, however, is usually small and minimally displaced.

Aviator's astragalus (an old word for the talus) is a fracture of the neck of the talus due to a plantar force which drives the talar neck into the anterior lip of the tibia. Any fractures or injuries causing complete dislocation of the talus are associated with avascular necrosis of the proximal fragment. This should be suspected in follow up films when the density of the proximal fragment remains constant while the remainder of the bones of the ankle become osteoporotic because of hyperaemia.

> The higher the fibular fracture the more extensive the damage to the tibiofibular ligaments

Reasons for taking an ankle radiograph

Criteria for ankle radiography

The Royal College of Radiologists 1989 guidelines recommend selective radiographs in patients presenting with an ankle injury with one or more of the following signs:

Deformity, crepitus, or instability
Bruising or severe swelling
Moderate or severe pain on weight bearing
Point tenderness on palpation
Injury of tendon, vessel, or nerve
Suspected foreign body
Age

A radiograph is unlikely to show a fracture if the patient is able to continue with his or her activity, is able to bear weight with moderate ease, has no swelling or joint tenderness over the bone, and has no swelling over the anterior tibiofibular ligament

The decision when to radiograph an ankle depends on the clinical findings and the mechanism of injury. A higher index of suspicion and a lower threshold for radiological assessment is needed in elderly patients, who can sustain fractures with minimal trauma.

Types of view

Radiographic projections for ankle

Standard:
   Lateral (fig 2)
   Anteroposterior (fig 1)
 	
Additional:
   Mortice
   Oblique

The mortice view is a modified anteroposterior view with the foot internally rotated through 20°. When oblique views are indicated the ankle joint is rotated 45° internally and externally. Stress views and special techniques such as tenography, tomography, computed tomography, ultrasonography, and magnetic resonance imaging all have a role in investigating ligamentous tears but should not be undertaken without consultation with an experienced radiologist. Weight bearing radiographs are of little help.

Stress views taken under medical supervision help determine the extent of ligamentous injuries. However, these should not be performed until five to seven days after injury, when the pain and swelling have subsided. Such radiographs are contraindicated in the acute situation and in patients with a fracture.

System of radiological assessment

Criteria for fracture
Primary signs Breaks in the cortex of the bone Abnormal lucency or sclerosis in the medulla Abnormal alignment of the bone Abnormal shortening or lengthening *Secondary signs* Fat-blood levels in the adjacent joint (if the film is taken across the table with a horizontal beam) Fragments from parent bone Adjacent soft tissue swelling

A streak of high density in the trabecular bone is always abnormal and suggests an impacted fracture

Lateral view

We recommend using the ABCs system of radiographic interpretation.

Check the adequacy and quality of the radiograph

Check name, age, and sex of the patient, that the correct side has been radiographed, and that the correct region has been included. The malleoli should be superimposed on each other and the entire calcaneus and bones of the mid-foot, including the base of the fifth metatarsal, be visible. If the radiograph has been properly exposed, you should not need to use a bright light to see soft tissues.

Check alignment of bones—The malleoli are superimposed with the tibia articulating with the dome of the talus. The contiguous surfaces of the tibia and talus are smooth and symmetrical. The subtalar joint is visible.

Check bone margins and density—Follow the cortex of the bones of the ankle looking for any sudden changes in direction. Start by tracing down the posterior aspect of the tibia to the posterior aspect of the ankle joint. Follow the joint surface of the tibia anteriorly then, passing upwards, trace the anterior margin of the tibia. Look through the tibia to trace the surface of the fibula. Next trace the margins of the talus in a similar clockwise fashion. The margins are normally partly obscured in the anterior and posterior portions of the subtalar joint. Examine the internal density and structure of all the visible bones. The trabeculae in the medullary canal should be of uniform or gradually changing density.

Check the cartilage and joints—The contiguous surfaces of the talus and distal tibia should be smooth and symmetrical with the distal tibia lying on the posterior aspect of the dome of the talus.

Check soft tissues—Extracapsular soft tissue swelling about the ankle joint is often seen in trauma and is a non-specific sign that is usually not associated with bony injury. Anterior to the ankle joint a vertical soft tissue fat density is visible. This relates to the anterior aspect of the joint capsule. When a severe joint effusion is present the joint capsule bulges. Rupture of the Achilles' tendon may be seen in plain films, although it is usually detectable clinically if complete. If incomplete, ultrasonography or magnetic resonance imaging may be required for diagnosis.

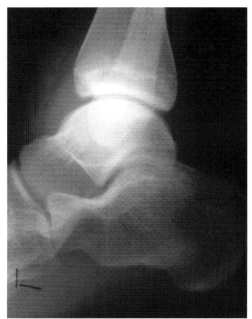

FIG 9—Ankle joint effusion. Note the displaced fat plane.

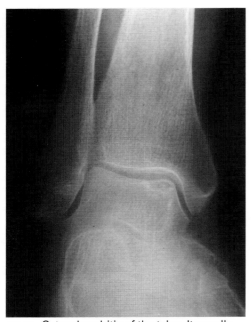

FIG 10—Osteochondritis of the talus. It usually occurs at the medial aspect of the superior surface and is identified as a separated piece of bone and associated cartilage.

Anteroposterior radiograph

Check the adequacy and quality of the radiograph—The anteroposterior radiograph of the ankle should show both malleoli and the talus (fig 1). The relation of the talus to the mortice cannot be optimally assessed. (This requires the mortice view, in which there is 20° internal rotation.)

Check alignment of bones—The talus should be in the mortice.

Check bone margins and density—Follow the scheme described for the lateral projection—that is, examine the cortical margins in a clockwise fashion then inspect the internal bony structure.

Check the cartilage and joints—In this projection the distal tibiofibular joint is obscured by the superimposed portions of the tibia and fibula. The distance between the contiguous surfaces of the talus and distal tibia/fibula should be equal in its medial, superior, and lateral aspects (fig 7). Check the distance of the distal tibiofibular joint looking for diastasis. Check there is no compression fracture of the tibial plate or osteochondritis tali.

Check soft tissues—Extracapsular soft tissue swelling about the ankle joint is often seen in trauma. It is a non-specific sign and is not usually associated with bony injury.

Catches to avoid

Acute osteomyelitis

Acute bone infection produces swelling and irregular demineralisation of the affected bone but demineralisation is often difficult to detect. Periosteal new bone formation also occurs, but these bony changes are not evident for 10-14 days. The diagnosis is therefore initially clinical. Specialist advice should be sought early if this condition is suspected.

Summary
Check the adequacy and quality
Check alignment of bones
Check bone margins and density
Check the cartilage and joints
Check soft tissues

The os trigonum is a common normal variant of the talus and is due to a separate ossification centre arising from the posterior tubercle. The appearance may resemble an old ununited fracture fragment. However, it is triangular, well corticated, in a classic location, and usually bilateral, which enables it to be distinguished from a fracture.

Fibrous cortical defects are the most commonly seen benign lesions of long bones and are usually identified incidentally in radiographs taken for another reason. The defect is limited to the cortex, commonly found at the metaphysis, but may be located in the diaphysis as the bone grows. The lesion is well corticated (sclerotic margins) and usually does not produce signs or symptoms.

Transverse, sclerotic, linear lines located at the metaphysis of growing long bones are due to short periods of growth arrest and have no clinical importance (fig 5). They may be confused with compression fractures, but again as with ossification centres these lines are usually bilateral.

KNEE

P Sanville, D A Nicholson, P A Driscoll

Most knee injuries are confined to the soft tissues and are invisible in plain radiographs

The exposed position of the knee and its functional demands make it one of the most vulnerable joints to injury, especially in athletes. In most cases, however, the plain films look normal and clinical examination does not show any disruption of ligaments. This article describes the common types of bony injury that are found and advises how to assess plain radiographs.

Important anatomical considerations

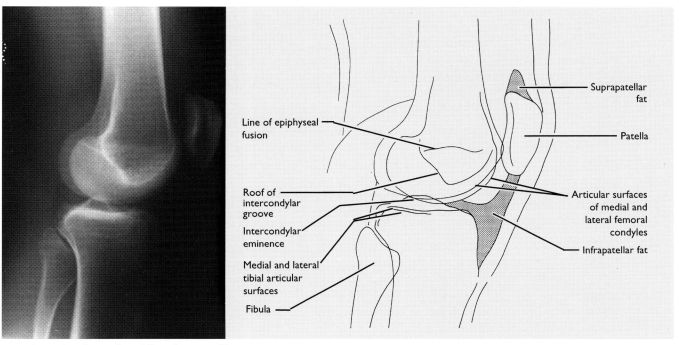

FIG 1—Lateral radiograph and line diagram of knee.

Fractures of the fibular neck and head may be associated with damage to the common peroneal nerve and collateral ligament complex and may be part of a pronation-lateral rotation ankle injury.

The arterial blood supply can be compromised in fractures near the adductor canal and popliteal fossa because of impingement of fracture fragments. Tibial and fibular fractures can cause compression of vessels because of haematoma in the leg compartments.

Adult

The knee is a synovial joint formed by the femoral condyles articulating with the tibial condyles (figs 1 and 2). The patella lies within the quadriceps tendon. The posterior surface of this sesamoid bone has a steep sloping medial articulating facet and a shallower lateral facet for articulation with the femoral condyles.

The common peroneal nerve runs close to the neck of the fibula and is prone to injury. Posteriorly, the popliteal artery is closely related to the tibial plateau and may be damaged by fracture fragments or in dislocation of the knee.

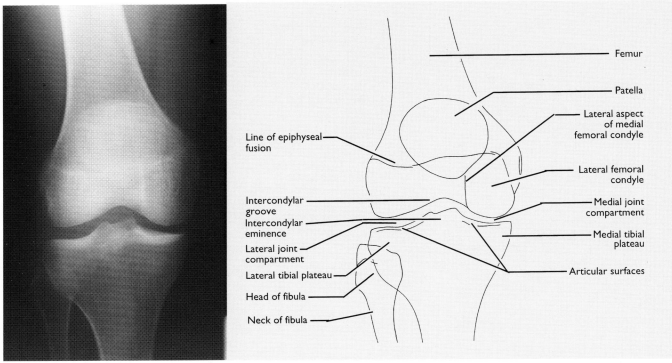

FIG 2—Anteroposterior radiograph and line diagram. Note the slight reduction of the medial joint compartment.

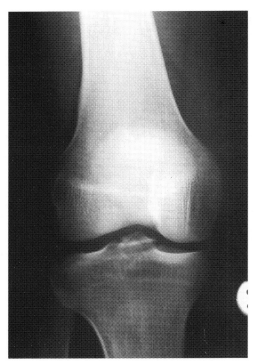

FIG 3—Avulsion fracture of the intercondylar eminence.

There is a complex arrangement of ligaments around the knee including the medial, lateral, and cruciate ligaments. Part of the lateral ligament complex is attached to the fibular head. Injury to any of these complexes causes instability of the knee. The anterior cruciate ligament is attached to the medial tibial spine so avulsion fractures of this spine or of the base of the intercondylar eminence are important. The posterior cruciate attaches to the posterior aspect of the intercondylar region away from the lateral spine. An avulsion fracture of this spine is therefore less important.

The menisci help the smooth movement, including rotation of the knee joint, and are not normally visible in plain films. There are a large number of bursae around the knee, not all of which communicate with the joint cavity. Effusions are commonly seen in the suprapatellar bursa behind the quadriceps tendon. As there is little overlying soft tissue, fractures of the tibia and fibula tend to be compounded.

Children

The distal femoral and proximal tibial epiphyses are present from birth until 18-20 years. The non-ossified cartilage overlying the femoral epiphysis is visible in the lateral film as an irregular soft tissue density around the epiphysis. The distal femoral epiphysis may be seen to be cleft.

The patella starts to ossify between the ages of 3 and 6 years. Several ossification centres may fail to fuse, simulating fractures. A horizontally bifid patella is a normal variant best seen in the lateral film, which usually goes on to unite.

Assessment of the physis

Look carefully for widening or compression, which may affect part or all of the physis. Compression fractures can be very subtle. Injury to the physis can be associated with stunted growth.

Mechanisms of injury

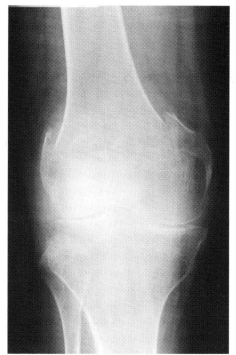

FIG 4—Impacted comminuted supracondylar fracture. Note the fracture lines extending up the femoral shaft.

Femur—distal two thirds

Fractures of the femoral shaft usually result from considerable force. The quadriceps and hamstring muscles tend to produce shortening and displacement of the fractures and there can be considerable loss of blood. Serious rotation of the distal fragment is easily overlooked unless the whole femur is surveyed in two projections.

Supracondylar fractures in adults often result in rotation of the distal fragment because of the pull of the gastrocnemius muscle. In children, these fractures are usually minimally displaced.

Femoral condylar fractures can be displaced or undisplaced and affect one or both condyles. If the fracture is completely intra-articular the bones may not reunite because the synovial fluid interferes with the organisation of the haematoma. Severely comminuted condylar fractures may be associated with a spiral fracture of the distal femur.

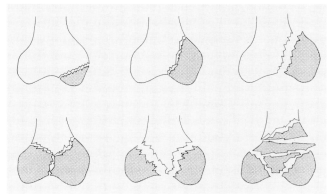

FIG 5—Fractures of the femoral condyle

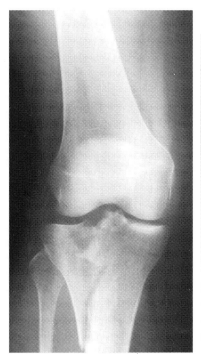
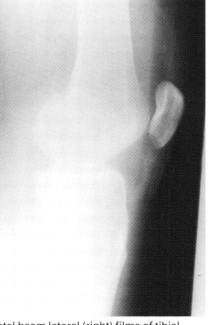

FIG 6—Anteroposterior (left) and horizontal beam lateral (right) films of tibial plateau fracture due to valgus strain. The large lipohaemarthrosis is due to a comminuted, displaced fracture of the lateral tibial plateau affecting the intercondylar eminence. Note that the fibular head is intact implying disruption of the tibiofibular ligament.

Tibia and fibula—proximal third

A fracture of the lateral tibial condyle commonly results from severe valgus stress (such as being hit by a car bumper). With further force the fibular neck fractures and the medial collateral and cruciate ligaments tear causing medial subluxation of the tibia. Bicondylar fractures may be seen. If there is a severely depressed fracture of the tibial plateau and no fibular fracture then disruption of the proximal tibiofibular joint has occurred.

Isolated silent fractures of the proximal fibula are seen in patients who have had parachute accidents. These are often misdiagnosed as a soft tissue injury clinically.

Osgood-Schlatter disease is due to recurrent contraction of the quadriceps in teenage athletes. Plain radiographs may show soft tissue swelling over the tibial tubercle, which is raised away from the tibia. These findings are non-specific and the disease should be diagnosed only in conjunction with the clinical findings of pain, tenderness, and swelling.

Patella

When the patella is fractured by direct violence a femoral shaft fracture and posterior dislocation of the hip may also occur. This is seen typically in patients who hit the dashboard in car accidents.

Fractures of the patella may be vertical, horizontal, or comminuted. Vertical fractures are usually stable but distraction of the fragments is common in horizontal fractures. If the bones are undisplaced in the initial film, weekly follow up for three weeks is advisable to detect late separation.

Dislocation of the patella often recurs. It is seen typically in teenage girls and always occurs laterally because of the flat lateral condyle and the oblique pull of the quadriceps muscle. It is caused by muscular contraction or a blow to the medial patella. There are several predisposing conditions that can be assessed in plain films.

In complete lateral dislocation the patella will lie lateral and parallel to the lateral femoral epicondyle. Minor degrees of subluxation can be seen. An osteochondral avulsion fracture from the lateral femoral condyle or the medial patella in the skyline view suggests a previous patellar dislocation.

Dislocation of the knee

Dislocation of the knee is rare because the surrounding ligments are strong. However, it can occur with relatively trivial trauma. The tibia is usually displaced anteriorly but posterior, lateral, medial, and rotational dislocation can occur. The ligament and joint capsule are always severely damaged, and a fracture of the proximal tibia and vascular damage are often present.

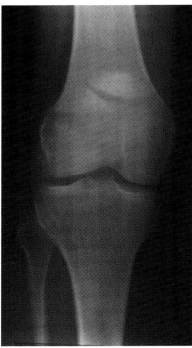

FIG 7—Anteroposterior film of horizontal patellar fracture showing slight separation of the fragments. Late separation may occur.

Soft tissue injuries

Most knee injuries are confined to the soft tissues and are not visible in plain radiographs. A varus stress to the knee damages the lateral ligament complex. There may be an associated avulsion fracture of the head of the fibula or the proximal tibia (fig 8).

Types of view

Knee

All patients with knee injuries should have an anteroposterior and lateral view of the distal femur, proximal tibia, and fibula. A horizontal beam lateral film is essential in all trauma patients to detect lipohaemarthrosis (fig 6). The initial plain film findings and clinical examination are used to determine which other views are required.

A tunnel view of the intercondylar notch is useful for assessing osteochondral fractures, the tibial spines, and intra-articular loose bodies as superimposition of the femoral condyles is reduced. Frontal oblique views in internal and external rotation help to evaluate the tibial plateau and spines.

Distal femur, proximal tibia, and fibula

Anteroposterior and lateral views of the whole femur are needed to assess angulation, displacement, and rotation of the distal femur accurately.

Fractures of the proximal third of the fibula can be associated with a fracture of the distal tibia or with rupture of the distal tibiofibular ligaments and the interosseous membrane. The anteroposterior and lateral views should therefore include the knee and the ankle if clinically indicated.

System of radiological assessment

The medullary bone
Look for subtle lucent fracture lines or discontinuity in the trabecular pattern. Stress fractures of the proximal tibia appear as a thickened sclerotic transverse band and a lucent line may extend through part of the cortex.

Skyline view of patella
In this view the patella should fit snugly in the intercondylar notch with equal joint space on its medial and lateral surfaces.

Subcutaneous emphysema
In perforating injuries or compound fractures air in the soft tissues of joint spaces can cause areas of increased lucency.

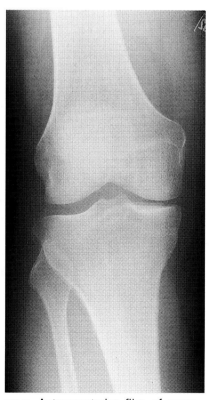

FIG 8—Anteroposterior film of varus strain injury showing lateral widening of the joint space and an avulsion fracture of the lateral tibial condyle.

Lateral projection

Follow the ABCs system of assessment.

Check the adequacy and quality of the radiograph—The fibular head overlaps the posterior tibia and the femoral condyles are superimposed. The radiographic density should allow the soft tissues, and particularly the suprapatellar pouch, to be evaluated.

Check alignment of bones—With the knee extended the patella lies anterior to the proximal portion of the femoral condyles. The patella may be invisible if there is complete lateral dislocation as it becomes superimposed over the lateral femoral condyle. The femoral condyles should articulate with the tibial plateau.

Check bone margins and density—Starting with the distal femur, trace around the cortical margin ensuring that there is no discontinuity, particularly in the supracondylar area. Trace the tibial cortex checking for a minimally displaced plateau fracture. This will appear either as an area of local sclerosis due to impaction or as a step defect. Trace the margin of the patella. Vertical fractures of the patella are usually undisplaced and invisible in the lateral film. Horizontal patellar fractures should be visible.

Cartilage and joints—The patellar femoral joint space should be visible, although slight overlap by a femoral condyle is normal. Meniscal tears are not visible in plain radiographs but an associated effusion may be seen.

Check soft tissues—An area of increased lucency due to fat is usually seen behind the quadriceps and prepatellar tendon. Joint effusions in the prepatellar pouch appear as a tongue of soft tissue density extending superiorly from the patellar-femoral joint into this lucent area. The patella will be displaced anteriorly and tilted inferiorly by a large effusion.

Anteroposterior projection

Check the adequacy and quality of the radiograph—The film should be centred on the joint space and the lateral tibia and the head of the fibula should overlap slightly. The patella should just be visible in the midline projected over the intercondylar notch.

Check alignment of bones—The femoral condyles should sit on the tibial condyles. The patella should lie in the midline. Dislocation of the patella will be seen in profile lateral to the lateral femoral epicondyle. Vertical patellar fractures may be visible superimposed over the dense femoral condyle.

Check bone margins and density—Starting with the most proximal part of the femur, trace the cortical margin clockwise. Repeat this for the tibia, paying particular attention to the tibial plateau. Undisplaced fractures cause a small step defect in the dense white line of the arttticular surface. Check that the medial and lateral tibial spines are intact. Look for small avulsion fractures at the site of insertion of the medial and lateral collateral ligaments. Observe the neck of the fibula for a fracture. Examine the patella.

Cartilage and joints—Assess the joint spaces between the femoral and tibial condyles. The medial and lateral compartments should be equal in height. Note the double contour of the medial tibial plateau—the distal line is the articular surface.

Check soft tissues—Look for evidence of subcutaneous emphysema or any foreign body. Chondrocalcinosis due to calcification of the menisci produces a thin line of calcification parallel to the tibial condyles, especially in older patients with osteoarthritis.

Catches to avoid

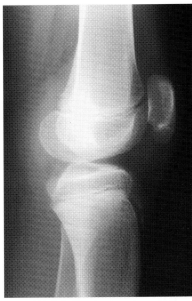

FIG 9—Well defined sclerotic margins between the patella and an accessory ossification centre in a 12 year old child. Note the normal epiphyses and tibial tubercle apophysis.

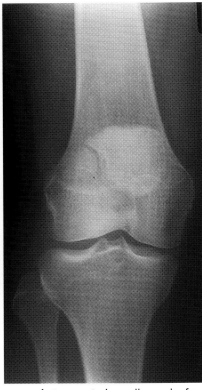

FIG 10—Anteroposterior radiograph of a bipartite patella showing the separate fragment in the typical site.

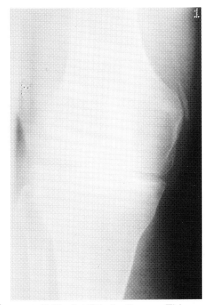

FIG 9—Pelligrini-Stieda disease. This should be distinguished from an acute avulsion injury.

The fabella is commonly seen lying in the lateral head of gastrocnemius, posterolateral to the knee.

The normal fat pad lying immediately posterior to the patellar tendon may look like a small lipohaemarthrosis in the lateral view but it will be visible in a film taken with a vertical *x* ray beam, unlike a true lipohaemarthrosis.

The patella may be bipartite. In this case a separate upper outer portion with well defined rounded margins is seen in the anteroposterior and skyline patellar views. Less commonly the patella is segmented in up to four pieces.

In children the anteroposterior view may show developmental lucent stripes on the medial aspect of the distal femoral epiphysis which simulate fractures.

An ununited accessory ossification centre of the fibular head will have a smooth corticated margin unlike a fracture. A thin line of ossification may also be seen in the medial collateral ligament next to the insertion point on the medial femoral epicondyle. This is caused by an old avulsion injury of this ligament with subsequent calcification within the subperiosteal haematoma (Pelligrini-Stieda disease) (fig 10).

Summary

Diagnostic quality

Alignment of bones
 Femur: tibia
 Patella

Bone margins and density
 Femur, tibia, patella, fibula

Cartilage and joints
 Femorotibial
 Patellar-femoral

Soft tissues
 Effusions
 Lipohaemarthrosis
 Chondrocalcinosis
 Surgical emphysema
 Foreign bodies

HIP

P Sanville, D A Nicholson, P A Driscoll

The hip joint is a common site for trauma in adults and damage to the hip may be associated with injuries to the rest of the pelvis, the femur, and the knee. This chapter describes a system of assessment to help interpret hip radiographs.

Important anatomical considerations

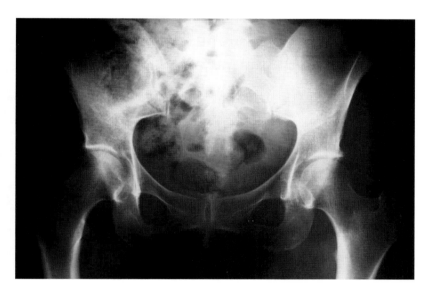

Adult

The strong hip joint capsule and the surrounding large muscle bulk prevent dislocation except in severe trauma. More commonly the hip is fractured with a resulting high incidence of avascular necrosis of the femoral head, complicating intracapsular fractures, and epiphyseal injuries. The trochanteric apophyses are the insertion points for the gluteus medius (greater trochanter) and iliopsoas (lesser trochanter) muscles and are prone to avulsion in athletic adolescents. In malignant disease the proximal femur, particularly the subtrochanteric region, is a common site for metastases and pathological fracture (fig 2).

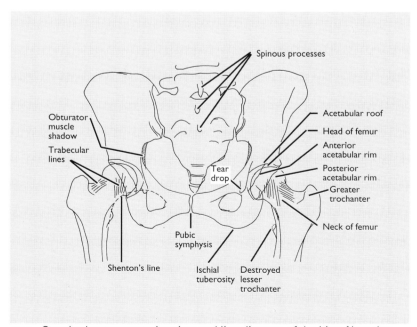

Children

The proximal capital femoral epiphysis is present from the age of 3 months until 18-20 years, with double epiphyseal ossification centres being common. Although asymmetry, irregular contour, and notching of the epiphyses can be normal variants in young children, a smaller epiphysis or any asymmetry in children with symptomatic hips may indicate injury. Flattening of the epiphysis is abnormal.

FIG 1—Standard anteroposterior view and line diagram of the hips. Note that the left lesser trochanter is destroyed by a metastasis.

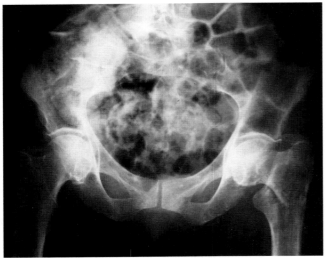

FIG 2—Left intertrochanteric pathological fracture. Note the large lucent trochanteric metastasis and disruption of Shenton's line.

The metaphysis has a rich blood supply and is a common site for osteomyelitis and consequently septic arthritis.

Mechanisms of injury

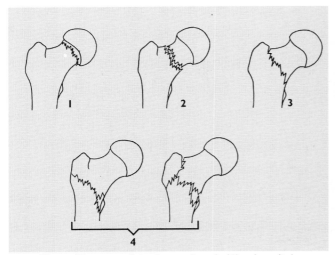

FIG 3—Sites of fracture of the femoral neck: (1) subcapital-intracapsular (most common site); (2) transcervical-intracapsular; (3) intertrochanteric-extracapsular fracture line along base of neck; (4) pertrochanteric-extracapsular without and with extension into proximal shaft as a spiral fracture.

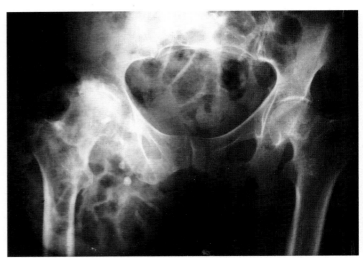

FIG 4—Left subcapital fracture. Note the upward displacement of the femur and abnormal Shenton's line. There is severe osteoarthritis of the right hip and a massive right inguinal hernia containing small bowel loops.

Femoral neck fractures

These fractures are seen most commonly in elderly osteopenic women after a fall. They also occur in men under 60 years after industrial accidents.

There are four sites of fracture (fig 3). Fractures may be intracapsular or extracapsular and are usually visible in the anteroposterior film as a lucent line. Pertrochanteric fractures are commonly comminuted with displacement of the lesser trochanter.

In children considerable violence is needed to fracture the neck of the femur. In transepiphyseal fractures the capital epiphysis is separated from the metaphysis and dislocated out of the acetabulum, often resulting in avascular necrosis.

Fractured neck of femur in children

Delbet classification:

Type 1—Transepiphyseal (avascular necrosis usually follows)

Type 2—Transcervical (avascular necrosis common if displaced)

Type 3—Cervicotrochanteric

Type 4—Pertrochanteric

Complications of hip dislocation

Slipped femoral epiphysis

Sciatic nerve palsy

Femoral nerve or artery compression (anterior dislocation)

Failed reduction and recurrent dislocation

Avascular necrosis of the femoral head

Osteoarthritis

Myositis ossificans

In severe trauma fractures of the patella and femoral shaft, neck, or head often occur in combination with central dislocation of the hip

---

Dislocation

The femoral head can be dislocated anteriorly, posteriorly, or centrally. Central dislocation occurs when the femoral head impacts through the acetabulum because of a sideways fall, a blow to the greater trochanter, or a fall from a height on to the feet. Falling on to the feet is often associated with a fracture of the anterior or posterior pelvic columns (see chapter on pelvis). Posterior dislocation may result from a blow to the lumbar spine—for example, from falling masonry—with the hip flexed. In patients who have hit a car dashboard dislocation of the hip is associated with a fracture of the femoral shaft or patella.

Slipped upper femoral epiphysis (adolescent coxa vara)

In this condition the femoral neck moves proximally and externally rotates on the unfused epiphysis. It is bilateral in 20% of cases and occurs in overweight, hypogonadal, or tall thin adolescents. Pain, sometimes referred to the knee, or limp is a common presenting symptom. Both hips should be evaluated. Early slip is best assessed in the lateral film (fig 5).

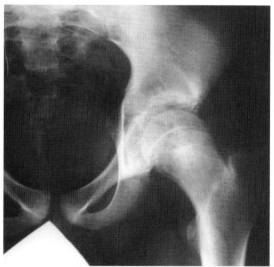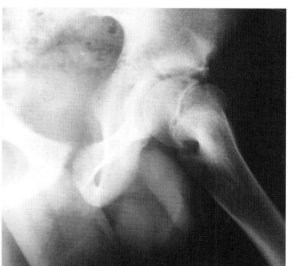

FIG 5—Radiographs of a 13 year old boy with an acutely painful left hip due to slipped upper femoral epiphysis. Left: anteroposterior coned film—the slip is not apparent. Note gonad protection. Right: oblique view of left hip. The femoral neck has slipped proximally over the epiphysis, which remains in the acetabulum and externally rotated resulting in a prominent lesser trochanter and superimposed greater trochanter.

Types of view

Radiographic views of the hip

Standard:
  Anteroposterior (fig 1)
  Cross table lateral (fig 8)

Additional
  Frog leg lateral
  Oblique (fig 5)

Routine radiographic examination should include an anteroposterior view of the whole pelvis (fig 1), which allows comparison between both hips, and a lateral view of the symptomatic joint if an abnormality is seen in the anteroposterior view or if slipped epiphysis is suspected.

Coned oblique views can be taken to assess acetabular fractures, undisplaced femoral neck fractures, and trochanteric fractures. The frog leg lateral film is useful in children. It shows the femoral head and neck in a position between the anteroposterior and the standard lateral projection.

Anteroposterior and lateral views of the femoral shaft and knee are indicated when there is a history of severe trauma or when clinical findings suggest more than one fracture site. Gonad protection should always be used in children and adults of reproductive age, providing it will not obscure a fracture.

System of radiological assessment

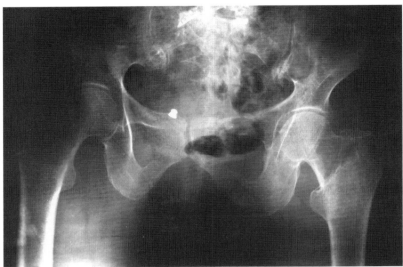

FIG 6—Undisplaced left pertrochanteric fracture. Note the lucent line extending into a break in the cortex of the greater trochanter. An air gun pellet is lying in the abdominal wall.

Follow the ABCs system of adequacy alignment, bones, cartilage and joints, and soft tissue.

Anteroposterior projection

Check the adequacy and quality of the radiograph—The anteroposterior film centred just above the pubic symphysis should include the whole pelvis and proximal third of the femur. The lumbar spinous processes, coccyx, and pubic symphysis will form a vertical straight line in a non-rotated film.

Check alignment of bones—The medial half of the femoral head overlaps the posterior acetabular rim. The curve of the lower border of the superior pubic ramus and the inferior aspect of the neck of the femur should form a smooth arc (Shenton's line).

> The plain film usually shows no abnormality in children presenting with an irritable hip. However, orthopaedic referral is mandatory

Check bone margins and density—Trace around the margin of the proximal femur, starting at the inferior aspect of the medial femoral cortex and checking for any disruption of the cortical line, particularly around the neck or trochanters (fig 6). In patients who can bear weight, carefully examine the trabecular lines and cortical margins of the femoral neck in a coned anteroposterior film to detect undisplaced fractures. Undisplaced femoral neck fractures will have a discontinuity in the trabecular lines, with an associated linear increase in density when impacted (figs 7 and 8). Check the cortical lines of the acetabular joint surface and posterior and anterior rim. Both hips should be symmetrical.

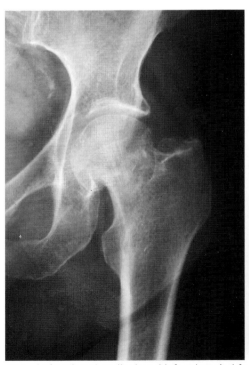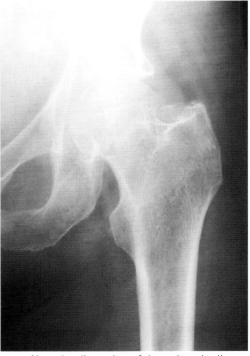

FIG 7—Left: missed undisplaced left subcapital fracture. Note the disruption of the trabecular lines. Right: same patient three weeks later. Ill defined areas of sclerosis are seen in the fracture line due to impaction. Shenton's line is now disrupted.

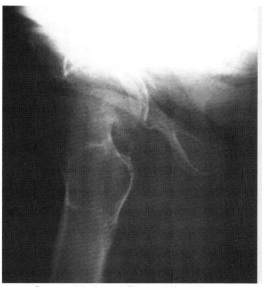

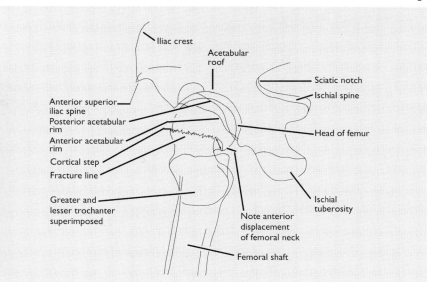

FIG 8—Cross table lateral film and line diagram of the left hip (of the same patient as in figure 7). The femoral neck is displaced anteriorly and impacted into the head of femur.

Diagram labels:
- Iliac crest
- Acetabular roof
- Sciatic notch
- Ischial spine
- Anterior superior iliac spine
- Posterior acetabular rim
- Anterior acetabular rim
- Head of femur
- Cortical step
- Fracture line
- Greater and lesser trochanter superimposed
- Note anterior displacement of femoral neck
- Ischial tuberosity
- Femoral shaft

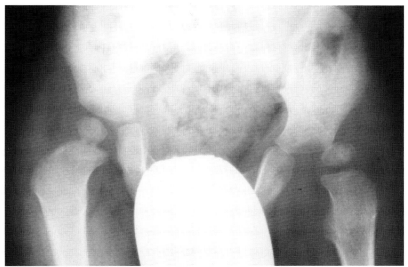

FIG 9—Acute septic arthritis of the left hip in a 1 year old boy. The left femoral capital epiphysis is greatly displaced out of the acetabulum by an effusion and is starting to disintegrate. Emergency drainage is required.

Cartilage and joints—In children widening of the joint space between the tear drop and the cortex of the femoral head may be seen in joint effusions (fig 9). A difference greater than 2 mm between the two sides is clinically important. Check that the physis (growth plate) is not widened or compressed (Salter-Harris types 1 and 5 fractures).

Check soft tissues—Because of the large muscle mass around the hip, soft tissue injuries are not visible in plain radiographs. Air or a metallic foreign body will be visible after a penetrating injury. If air is seen outlining the femoral head or acetabulum the joint capsule has been breached.

The lateral projection

Check the adequacy and quality of the radiograph.—The cross table lateral film should include the acetabulum, the ischial spine and tuberosity, and the proximal femur. The trochanters overlap. In the frog leg lateral film, the greater trochanter should be projected over the neck of femur.

Check alignment of bones—The femoral neck lies anteverted about 30° to the femoral shaft. Check that the entire metaphysis is covered by epiphysis in children and adolescents. In slipped upper femoral epiphysis the centre of the femoral neck metaphysis lies anterior to its normal position over the central epiphysis (figs 4 and 5). In patients with dislocated hips the cross table lateral film will define whether dislocation is anterior or posterior.

Check bone margins and density—Trace around the margins of the femur and then the acetabulum and ischium. If a dislocation is present look for acetabular fragments. These are usually displaced in the same direction as the femoral head.

Check soft tissues

Acetabular fractures

- Are easily missed in the anteroposterior film and can simulate normal variants
- Can be associated with an isolated superior pubic ramus fracture
- May be complicated by sciatic nerve palsy and severe intrapelvic haemorrhage

Catches to avoid

Summary

Adequacy of radiograph

Alignment of bones

Bone margins and density
   Fractures

Cartilage and joints

Soft tissues

Accessory ossification centres, recognised by their corticated margins, are common around the acetabular margins and may simulate fractures when partially fused in adolescence. They may persist into adult life. Acetabular roof notches and roof asymmetry are recognised normal variants. Symmetrical protrusion of the acetabular roofs medially is common in 4-12 year olds.

Hypertrophic changes of the femoral head or inferior aspect of the neck may simulate fractures. Skin folds are superimposed over the intertrochanteric region (they extend past the outer cortical margins; this differentiates them from fractures).

In early childhood the trabecula of the femoral neck may produce a striated pattern or unusual lucencies simulating osteomyelitis.

CHEST

D W Hodgkinson, B R O'Driscoll, P A Driscoll, D A Nicholson

> Get a posteroanterior film whenever possible

Chest radiographs are commonly requested and taken in accident and emergency departments and in many emergency situations in hospital. This chapter details the types of urgent chest radiograph available and provides a systematic method for interpreting films. It also describes the common emergency conditions requiring chest radiographs and the relevant radiological signs.

Important anatomical consideration

The plain chest radiograph allows assessment of the heart, lungs, mediastinum, and chest wall. You need to be familiar with the main anatomical features seen in posteroanterior and lateral chest radiographs together with common normal variations.

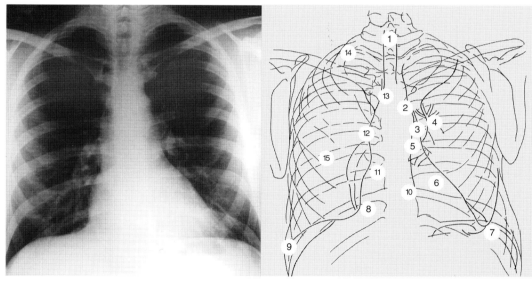

1) Trachea
2) Aortic knuckle
3) Left pulmonary artery
4) Left hilum
5) Left atrial appendage
6) Left ventricle
7) Left hemidiaphragm
8) Right cardiophrenic angle
9) Right costophrenic angle
10) Right ventricle
11) Right atrium
12) Right hilum
13) Superior vena cava
14) Right first rib
15) Horizontal fissure

FIG 1—Normal posteroanterior chest radiograph with line diagram.

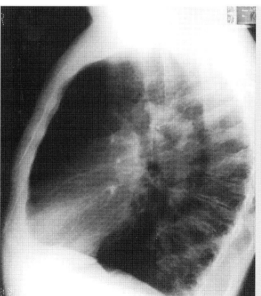
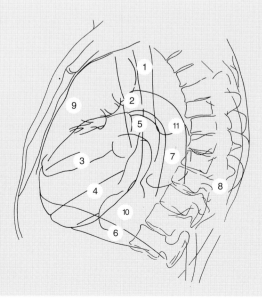

1) Trachea
2) Ascending aorta
3) Horizontal fissure
4) Oblique fissure
5) Hilar density
6) Diaphragms (right usually higher)
7) Descending thoracic aorta
8) Bones of dorsal spine are seen clearly in most films
9) Anterior cardiac window
10) Posterior cardiac window
11) Edge of scapula

FIG 2—Normal lateral chest radiograph with corresponding line diagram.

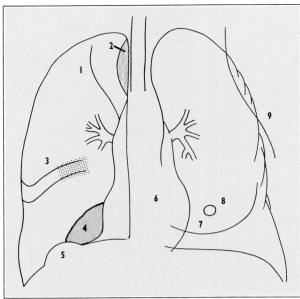

1) Azygous lobe (mistaken for bulla or pneumothorax)
2) Prominent brachiocephalic vessels (mistaken for right upper mediastinal mass or lymphadenopathy)
3) Calcified costal cartilages (mistaken for pleural or pulmonary lesions)
4) Pericardial cyst or fat pad (mistaken for cardiomegaly, tumour, or consolidation)
5) Diaphragmatic hump (mistaken for tumour or consolidation)
6) Unusual cardiac shape or apparent cardiomegaly may be caused by pectus excavatum with depressed sternum. (Confirmed by clinical examination and lateral radiograph (fig 4))
7) Asymmetrical breast shadows (mistaken for lower zone consolidation)
8) Prominent nipple shadow (mistaken for pulmonary nodule)
9) Loose folds of skin (especially in anteroposterior supine film). These may be mistaken for a pneumothorax but the loose skinfold can usually be followed outside the rib cage

FIG 3—Normal common variants.

Types of view

Potential pitfalls of the anteroposterior film

Cardiomegaly

Wide mediastinum

High diaphragms

Vague lower zone shadowing due to poor inspiration

Rotation artefacts

In the supine film:

Upper lobe blood diversion may be normal

Small pneumothorax may be missed (air collects anteriorly)

Pleural effusion may be missed (fluid collects posteriorly giving appearance of diffuse shadowing)

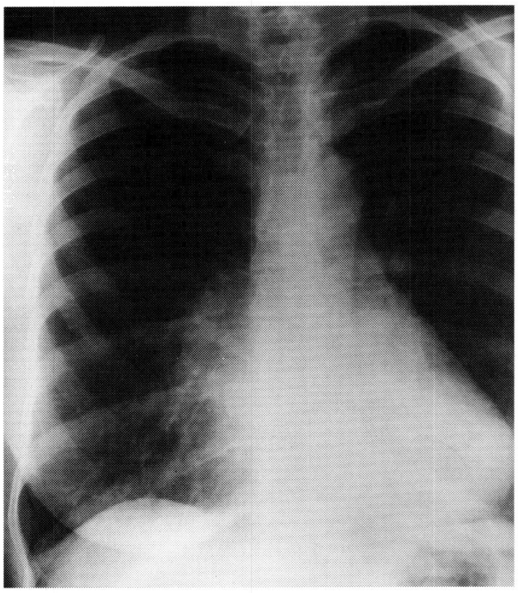

FIG 4—Posteroanterior film showing pectus excavatum and giving the impression of cardiomegaly. The cardiac shadow seems to shift to the left with loss of definition of the right heart border. The posterior ribs are horizontal and the anterior ribs vertical.

Though most patients require only one good quality film, other specialised views will be needed to identify some abnormalities.

Posteroanterior view—This film is taken in the radiology department. The patient stands with his or her anterior chest against the film cassette and the exposure is taken in full inspiration with the *x* ray source located 2 metres behind the patient. It is used for all cases unless the patient requires ongoing assessment, resuscitation, treatment, or monitoring.

Anteroposterior view—This view is usually requested for seriously ill patients with a life threatening condition that requires assessment, monitoring, or treatment in a resuscitation area. The film cassette is placed behind the patient, who sits or lies on the bed or trolley. A portable *x* ray machine is used. Non-essential medical and nursing staff leave the immediate area during exposure. There are several potential pitfalls that should be remembered when requesting and interpreting this film.

Lateral chest film—This view is rarely helpful in the emergency situation. It can, however, reveal abnormalities that are obscured by the heart or are hidden in the costophrenic recess in the posteroanterior film. It can also help localise an abnormality which has been identified in the posteroanterior or anteroposterior view. Remember that an extrathoracic foreign body may appear to be intrathoracic in a posteroanterior or anteroposterior view.

Lateral decubitus film—This is a posteroanterior chest film taken with the patient lying on his or her side (usually the abnormal side down). It can identify a small pleural effusion and differentiate this from pleural thickening. A subpulmonary haemothorax may become apparent with this view when the only abnormality seen in the posteroanterior film is a raised hemidiaphragm.

Sternal view—This is used to assess patients with suspected fractured sternum.

Rib views are rarely indicated because rib fractures are diagnosed from the clinical features. Remember that rib fractures may be associated with more important and serious chest injuries. Absence of rib fractures in a posteroanterior film does not exclude their presence or, more importantly, a serious intrathoracic injury.

The lateral chest radiograph is rarely helpful in acute conditions. However, it can localise abnormalities seen in the posteroanterior view

Expiration films may be used to show a small pneumothorax, but it is not necessary to request this view routinely because most pneumothoraces will be apparent in the posteroanterior inspiration film. Expiration films are occasionally requested to help establish a diagnosis of inhaled foreign body, when "gas trapping" may be seen.

Apical lordotic view—This is an oblique view that can show details of the lung apex which are usually hidden behind the clavicle and upper ribs. This technique is seldom indicated in the emergency situation.

System of radiological assessment

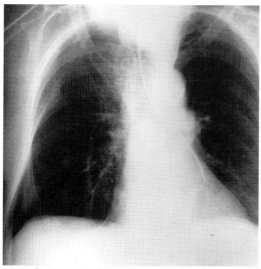

FIG 5—Posteroanterior radiograph of patient with feeding line in the left main bronchus.

First check the name and age of the patient together with the date on the radiograph.

Check the adequacy and technical quality of the film
Note the following:
Projection and exposure—Look at the mid-thoracic intervertebral discs; they should be clearly visible.
Posture—Supine or erect.
Rotation—Look at the spinous processes of the upper thoracic vertebrae. They should be central. Then inspect the medial end of both clavicles to ensure they are equidistant from the central spinous process.
Degree of inspiration—This affects the appearance of the lower zone vessels. They appear more prominent with poor inspiration. The right hemidiaphragm should reach the anterior end of the right sixth or seventh rib or the ninth rib posteriorly on full inspiration.

Check for any medical equipment
The position and presence of any invasive medical equipment (for example, endotracheal tubes, central venous cannulas) must be assessed (fig 5). The tip of the endotracheal tube should lie about 2 cm above the carina.

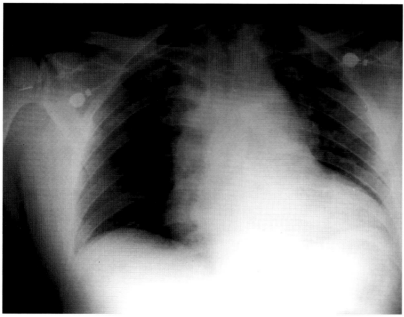

FIG 6—Semi-erect anteroposterior film showing evidence of a dissecting thoracic aorta with widening of the superior mediastinum (>10cm), blurring of the aortic outline, and opacification of the angle between the aorta and the left pulmonary artery (aortopulmonary bay). Depression of the left main bronchus should also be looked for.

Check the mediastinum
The mediastinum can be divided into upper, middle (hila), and lower (heart). The mediastinum should be central and its silhouette sharp. A double outline suggests pneumomediastinum. Further assessment depends on a knowledge of the normal anatomy and relative sizes of the mediastinal organs.

Start your inspection in the upper mediastinum on the left side. As you descend this border is interrupted by normal structures such as the aortic knuckle. Continue down the left border to the cardiophrenic angle, which should be acute and clear. Then follow the right border from the cardiophrenic angle back up to the upper mediastinum.

Next check the hila. These shadows are made up of pulmonary arteries and veins. The left hilum is usually 2 cm higher than the right. The heart is positioned with about one third of its diameter to the right and two thirds to the left of the spinous processes. A low diaphragm will cause a right shift and a high diaphragm a left shift. The heart's full diameter should be less than half of the internal thoracic diameter at its widest point (the cardiothoracic ratio).

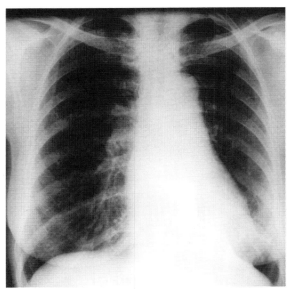

FIG 7—Increased wedge density behind the left heart shadow with loss of definition of the medial border of the left hemidiaphragm. The left hilum is not visible and there is crowding of the ribs representing generalised volume reduction in the left hemithorax. This represents left lower lobe collapse.

Common types of opacities in emergency radiographs

Large irregular opacities—for example, consolidation, collapse, carcinoma, pleural lesions, and chest wall lesions

Nodular opacities—single or multiple. In patients older than 45 years single nodules are most commonly due to bronchogenic tumours and multiple nodules to metastatic tumours

Ring shadows—for example, large bullae must be distinguished from a pneumothorax by their ring shadow or capsule

Linear and band shadows—for example, Kerley's B lines. These represent dilated lymphatic channels which become visible when the pulmonary arterial wedge pressure is >25 mm Hg. They are short, straight, peripheral lines that end at right angles against the pleura and are usually horizontal, <1 mm thick, and <2 cm long

Check the diaphragms

Examine the diaphragms specifically. Look for clear cardiophrenic and costophrenic angles. In 95% of normal subjects the right diaphragm is higher than the left by up to 3 cm.

The outline of the diaphragms is smoothly arcuate with the highest point medial to the midline of the hemithorax. Lateral peaking, particularly on the right, suggests a subpulmonary effusion or haemothorax in the appropriate clinical setting. Loss of clarity of the margin of the left diaphragm may indicate collapse or consolidation of the left lower lobe (fig 7).

Check the transradiancy of both lungs

Both lungs should be equal. Check them more specifically for fissures, vessels, and abnormal opacities. Look at the position, configuration, and thickness of fissures. Any fissure wider than hairline is considered abnormally thickened. The oblique fissure is normally seen in only the lateral view.

Both arteries and veins are visible, but it is not helpful to distinguish between them. They extend outwards from the mediastinum and disappear 2 cm or less from the lung margin. Carefully examine the apex of each lung field as apical lung lesions are commonly missed.

Check the bones

Examine the posterior, lateral, and anterior aspects of the ribs in detail, looking particularly for fractures and metastatic bone disease. Trace out laterally and anteriorly each rib from the posterior costochondral joint to where the rib joins the costochondral cartilage at the mid-clavicular line.

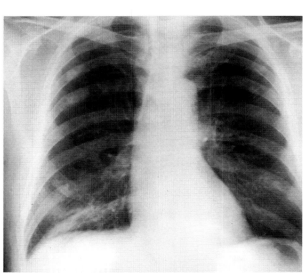

FIG 8—Opacification and consolidation in the right lower zone together with radiodense bone lesions in multiple ribs (right 5/6 and left 6/9). The patient had metastatic carcinoma of the prostate gland.

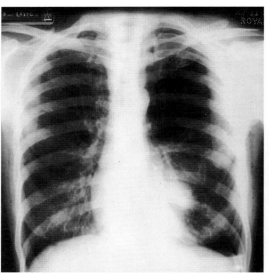
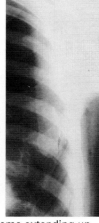

FIG 9—Left haemopneumothorax and surgical emphysema extending up the left of the chest (enlargement). The collapsed lung appears as an area of increased density obliterating the normal cardiac silhouette with increased transradiancy of the left upper and mid-zones.

Check both the upper and the lower borders of the rib. Then assess the clavicles and scapulae. Remember that information on both shoulder joints and the thoracic spine can be obtained from the chest film, but for proper assessment the appropriate special views must be obtained.

Check the extrathoracic soft tissues

Start at the top with the supraclavicular areas. Note any surgical emphysema, which is often seen in the cervical region. Continue down the lateral wall of the chest on each side. The assessment must include the breast shadows. Finally, check under the diaphragms for abnormal

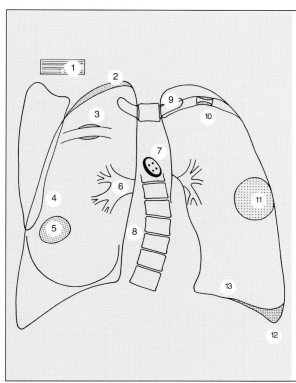

1) Wrong patient or wrong date
2) Small apical pneumothorax overlooked
3) Callus around old rib fracture misdiagnosed as pulmonary or pleural mass or rib tumour
4) Medial part of scapula may overlie lung field and be mistaken for a pneumothorax or pleural mass
5) Skin lesions (for example, a lipoma or sebaceous cyst) may be mistaken for an intrathoracic lesion
6) Prominent pulmonary arteries in emphysematous patients (due to pulmonary hypertension) may be mistaken for hilar tumour or nodes
7) Extraneous objects such as buttons or contents of pockets may be mistaken for intrathoracic lesions
8) Scoliosis or kyphosis may be overlooked. These make radiographs difficult to interpret as they commonly cause rotation and distortion of other chest structures
9) Costotransverse articulations (especially of upper ribs) may be mistaken for a fracture of the posterior rib
10) Lytic or sclerotic lesions of ribs are commonly overlooked
11) Large peripheral bullae may be mistaken for a pneumothorax
12) Scarring from old pleurisy or from thoracic surgery may cause blunting of the costophrenic angles and may be mistaken for an effusion. (The history and clinical signs should resolve this but if in doubt get a lateral decubitus view or an ultrasound scan)
13) Left mastectomy

FIG 10—Common mistakes.

Abnormalities associated with trauma

The common conditions seen in the accident and emergency department that require chest radiography can be divided into two types—those resulting from trauma and those from other causes.

Injuries associated with blunt thoracic trauma

Mechanism	Chest wall injury	Possible associated intrathoracic injury
Low energy transfer (direct blow)	Unilateral rib fracture	Pulmonary contusion
	Anterior sternal fracture	Cardiac contusion
High energy transfer (deceleration)	Chest wall may be intact	Ruptured aorta
		Cardiac contusion
	Bilateral rib fracture	Ruptured diaphragm
	Sternal fracture	Ruptured bronchus
Crush injury	Bilateral rib fractures with or without flail chest	Ruptured bronchus
		Cardiac contusion
	Ipsilateral rib fractures with or without flail chest	Pulmonary contusion
	Possible contralateral internal rib fracture	

There are three main mechanisms of chest trauma: low energy transfer (low velocity impact—for example, a kick), high energy transfer (high velocity impact—for example, a road traffic accident), and crush injury.

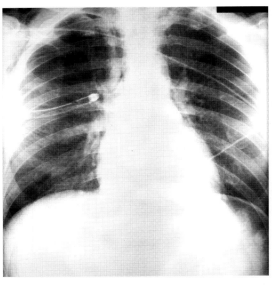

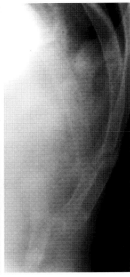

Rib fractures are best diagnosed clinically and are more common in high energy transfer and crush injuries (fig 11). Remember the chest film is requested to investigate the presence or absence of associated intrathoracic injuries.

Flail segment—This occurs when two or more ribs are fractured in two or more places or when the clavicle and first rib are similarly affected. It is associated with serious intrathoracic injury, especially pulmonary contusion, and may progress to respiratory failure.

FIG 11—Anteroposterior radiograph showing right intercostal drain, pneumomediastinum, and severe surgical emphysema (linear lucent lines in the right pectoral sheath overlying the right hemithorax and in the soft tissues). Rib fractures are seen in the enlarged detail

Signs of dissecting thoracic aorta

Widening of the superior mediastinum to >8 cm

Depression of the left main bronchus to an angle <40° with the trachea

Tracheal shift to the right

Blurring of the aortic outline

Obliteration of the medial aspect to the left upper lobe (pleural capping)

Opacification of the angle between the aorta and the left pulmonary artery

Lateral displacement of nasogastric tube in oesophagus

Causes of pneumomediastinum or surgical emphysema

Asthma

Ruptured oesophagus

Penetrating trauma

Ruptured bronchus

Aortic dissection—Ten per cent of patients with this condition survive to reach hospital They must be identified as soon as possible since a successful outcome depends on immediate identification and treatment. The diagnosis rests on a strong clinical suspicion, plain radiographic features, and ultimately arteriography.

Cardiac contusion is associated with crush and high energy transfer injuries. The chest radiograph may appear normal but there is usually evidence of disruption of the thoracic wall with or without pulmonary contusion.

Pulmonary contusion—Patchy consolidation is the early radiographic feature of this condition but this may underestimate the severity of the injury.

Ruptured major airway—This should be suspected in the presence of any of the following: pneumomediastinum, surgical emphysema in the neck, haemoptysis, collapse of a lung or lobe, pneumothorax with major air leak.

Ruptured diaphragm—This is more common on the left and should be suspected when there is a history of high energy transfer or crush injury with a bowel or stomach shadow in the thoracic cavity or an ill defined hemidiaphragm.

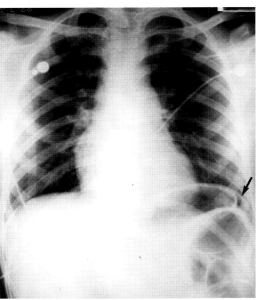

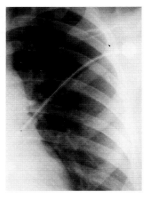

Penetrating chest trauma—The plain posteroanterior chest radiograph is the most important investigation (fig 12). Most penetrating wounds damage only the chest wall and underlying lung. Even the more serious injuries—for example, cardiac tamponade, transected aorta, lacerated diaphragm, and major airway injury—can be diagnosed by the mechanism of injury, the clinical findings, and a posteroanterior or anteroposterior chest radiograph. Remember that penetrating injuries to the neck and abdomen can affect the contents of the thoracic cavity. More specifically, globular enlargement of the cardiac silhouette may not be apparent in the plain film even in the presence of life threatening cardiac tamponade.

FIG 12—Small pneumoperitoneum caused by a stab wound to the left lower chest (arrow). An associated small pneumothorax is seen in the enlargement.

Non-trauma

When spontaneous thoracic aortic dissection is clinically suspected the patient should be further investigated by computed tomography or angiography

Radiological changes in pulmonary embolus

In many cases the chest radiograph appears normal

Early features which are occasionally seen:
  Raised hemidiaphragm
  Abnormally increased radiolucency due to reduced vessels distal to embolus (fig 16)
  Asymmetry of vessels compared with normal side
  Abrupt cut off or "rat tail" appearance of pulmonary vessels
Late features (commoner than early features):
  Pleural effusion
  Linear or wedge shaped shadows due to infarction of lung
  Occasionally infarcts may cavitate

Chest pain

A chest radiograph is not usually indicated in the early management of acute myocardial infarction and angina unless the diagnosis is in doubt. A patient with spontaneous thoracic aortic dissection may present with chest pain suggestive of acute myocardial infarction—a chest film may help but it is important to be aware of the pitfalls of interpreting an anteroposterior film. Occasionally the posteroanterior or the anteroposterior chest film, or both, may show clinically silent pulmonary oedema in patients with acute myocardial infarction.

Patients with severe acute central chest pain after vomiting who have a pneumomediastinum or increasing left sided pleural effusion on radiography may have a ruptured oesophagus. In acute pulmonary embolus the posteroanterior chest radiograph can show a variety of abnormalities but more commonly it appears normal. The combination of a breathless patient with or without chest pain and a normal posteroanterior chest radiograph does not exclude a pulmonary embolus. A common finding in a chest film is a hiatus hernia; this is not usually the cause of the patient's pain.

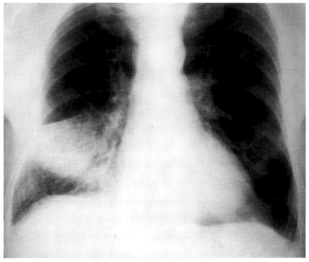

FIG 13—Right middle lobe pneumonia with a silhouette sign reducing the definition of the right heart border. There is slight volume loss in the middle lobe.

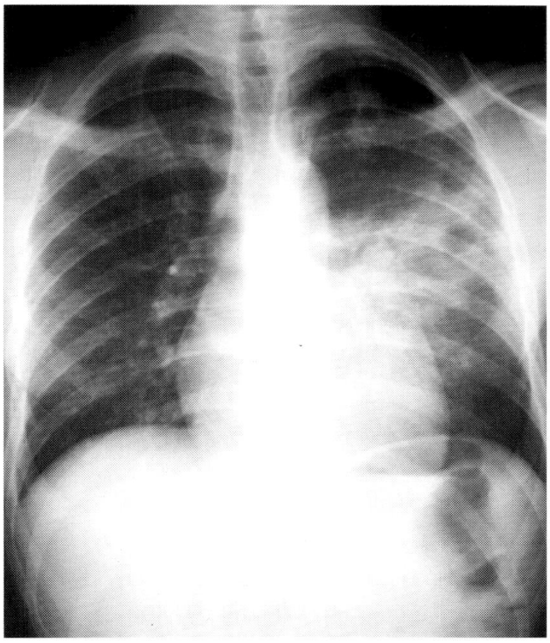

FIG 14—Consolidation in the left upper and mid-zones with cavitation in a patient with pulmonary tuberculosis.

Radiological features of pulmonary oedema

Early (pulmonary capillary wedge pressure <18-22 mm Hg):
  Upper lobe blood diversion
  Perihilar haze
  Peribronchial cuffing
  Vague increased density over lower lung fields

Late (pulmonary capillary wedge pressure >25 mm Hg):
  Kerley's A and B lines
  Extensive perihilar "bat's wing" shadowing
  Fluid passes into alveolar spaces producing diffuse poorly defined bilateral basal infiltrates

Chest infections

The chest radiograph can confirm a clinical diagnosis of pneumonia or pleural effusion (figs 13 and 14). The film usually appears normal in patients with acute asthma or exacerbated chronic obstructive pulmonary disease, but it is required to exclude conditions implicated in their aetiology or complications which will affect the patient's management—for example, pneumonic consolidation, pneumomediastinum, or pneumothorax. A chest radiograph is vital when an immunocompromised patient is thought to have an infection.

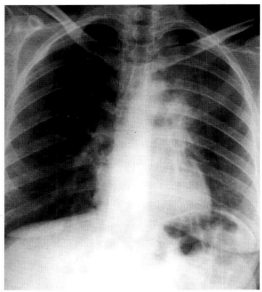

FIG 15—Left upper lobe collapse with the radiological signs of volume loss (raised left hemidiaphragm and raised left hilum) and loss of definition of the superior mediastinum on the left side (silhouette sign).

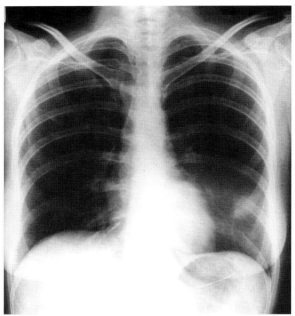

FIG 16—Abnormality in the transradiancy of the left lung field with a large irregular opacification in the left mid-zone. In this case it represented a pulmonary embolus.

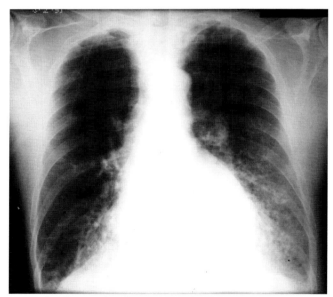

FIG 17—Cardiomegaly with severe pulmonary oedema. Peribronchial cuffing, well defined Kerley's B lines in the right lower zone, and bilateral alveolar shadowing are visible. Hyperinflation suggests pre-existing chronic obstructive pulmonary disease.

Haemoptysis

Look for evidence of lung cancer or tuberculosis (fig 14). A large tumour of the trachea or main bronchus may produce no radiological change until a lung suddenly collapses. Listen for stridor or monophonic wheeze. Don't forget pulmonary embolism.

Unexplained breathlessness

Look for a pneumothorax, evidence of heart failure, or unsuspected collapse of lobes or segments (figs 15 and 16). If the radiograph appears normal remember the possibility of neuromuscular disorders, pulmonary embolism, anaemia, central airway lesions (including radiolucent foreign bodies), and the hyperventilation syndrome.

Heart failure

The chest radiograph will usually confirm clinical suspicion of heart failure or show its severity. Radiological signs of heart failure precede clinical signs (fig 17).

Abdominal pain

Try to get an erect posteroanterior or anteroposterior chest film to look for free gas below the diaphragm (fig 18). Remember that cases of lower lobe pneumonia may present with abdominal pain.

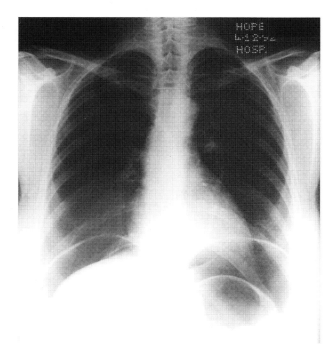

FIG 18—Large pneumoperitoneum with air under both diaphragms.

Neurological presentations and coma

Remember that any patient with dysphagia or a poor gag reflex is at risk of developing aspiration pneumonia. This is particularly relevant in unconscious patients. Initially there may be few radiological signs because aspiration pneumonia takes time to develop. This condition most commonly affects the right middle lobe (fig 13).

Inhaled foreign body

Metallic or bony foreign bodies may be seen in the routine radiograph. The lateral radiograph will show whether a coin is in the oesophagus or in the trachea. Inhaled organic material such as food is usually radiolucent, but a lobe or segment may have collapsed if the inhalation occurred some time previously. In acute aspiration air may be trapped in the affected lobe or segment, which may show up as hyperinflation with mediastinal shift to the normal side on the expiration film.

Useful radiological rules and signs

Pulmonary oedema

The radiographic changes are often worse than the clinical condition of the patient as fluid initially collects in the interstitium

The silhouette sign

Interfaces between lung and soft tissue structures will have clear margins in a chest radiograph provided that the interfaces are smooth and tangential to the x ray beam. If air in the lung at the interface is removed (for example, consolidation) the radiographic boundary will disappear (figs 13-15). This is known as the silhouette sign and it can be used to localise and identify both normal and abnormal structures.

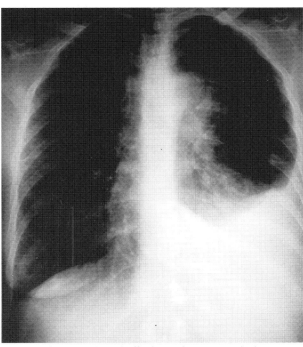

FIG 19—Left sided pleural effusion, a large mass lesion projected over the aortic knuckle, and a left mastectomy. This represents metastatic carcinoma of the breast.

Signs of consolidation (figs 13 and 14)

(1) Shadowing with ill defined margins due to piecemeal alveolar involvement. If the process comes up against a pleural surface the margin may be clearly defined (as in lobar pneumonia).

(2) No volume loss.

(3) Air bronchogram: normally intrapulmonary airways are invisible unless "end on" to the x ray beam, but if they pass through a zone of consolidation they become visible.

(4) Vascular changes: blood vessels are normally seen because their soft tissue density contrasts against air-containing lung, but with consolidation they become obscured.

Signs of pleural effusion (fig 19)

These signs are different in the erect and supine films.

Erect film—Homogenous opacification of the chest; obliteration of the costophrenic angle and the hemidiaphragm; the upper margin is concave to the lung and is higher laterally.

Supine film—Reduced transradiancy of the hemithorax due to dorsal pooling. The above signs are often absent.

Chest

Summary

Name, age, and date

Position of any invasive equipment

Mediastinum, including hila and size and shape of heart

Diaphragms, including costophrenic angles

Lung field abnormalities, including apices

Bones

Extrathoracic soft tissues

Signs of lobar collapse (fig 15)
  (1) Crowding of vessels and airways within the lobe.
  (2) Raised hemidiaphragm.
  (3) Shift of mediastinum, hilum, fissures, and other structures.
  (4) Compensatory hyperinflation.
  (5) Ribs close together.

ABDOMEN

D A Nicholson, P A Driscoll

Patients with abdominal symptoms account for a large proportion of people presenting as emergencies. Despite the development of other investigations plain film radiographs are still performed in most cases to look for intestinal obstruction or perforation. This article describes a systematic approach to the evaluation of abdominal radiographs and the next article will describe the different conditions commonly encountered.

> Plain radiographs remain the best method of detecting intestinal obstruction or perforation

Important anatomical considerations

> The abdominal radiograph lacks symmetry and has a wide variation in normal appearances, which makes interpretation difficult. Careful systematic interpretation is therefore essential

A thin layer of extraperitoneal fat lies in the lateral abdominal wall between the inner muscle layer (transverse abdominal muscle) and the parietal peritoneum. This produces a lucent shadow called the properitoneal line (flank stripe), which can extend from above the lateral margin of the liver to below the iliac crest. Similarly a thin layer of adipose tissue is often seen between the dome of the bladder and the pelvic peritoneum as a lucent line. These lines are not usually seen in infants or elderly patients because of scant adipose tissue. Normally the serosal surface of the ascending and descending colon is next to the parietal peritoneum, with a potential space (the paracolic gutter) between.

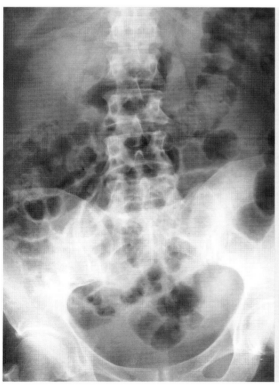
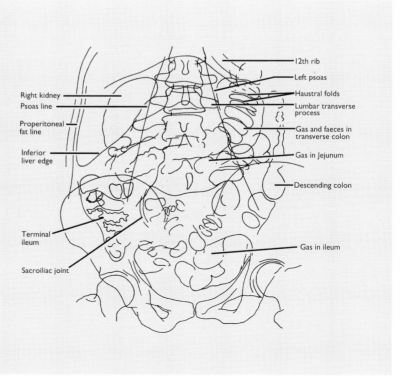

FIG 1—Normal supine abdominal radiograph and line diagram. A large amount of bowel gas is seen in the non-dilated small and large bowel because of air swallowing. The properitoneal fat line is clear on the right continuing lateral to the liver edge.

The supine abdominal radiograph is the standard projection.

Erect chest radiograph—The erect chest radiograph is a fundamental part of the examination of the acute abdomen as it is the most sensitive radiograph for detecting a small pneumoperitoneum. In addition, many intrathoracic conditions can mimic an acute abdominal emergency and elderly people may have coexisting chest disease.

Causes of chest disease mimicking an acute abdomen

Myocardial infarction
Pulmonary embolism
Pneumonia
Dissecting aortic aneurysm
Oesophageal disease

The erect abdominal radiograph adds little diagnostic information to the standard supine abdominal radiograph and erect chest radiograph and has been abandoned in many centres. It is occasionally needed to show the presence of air-fluid levels (see later). It must be remembered, however, that fluid levels are not pathognomonic of obstruction. A left lateral decubitus radiograph taken with a horizontal *x* ray beam is sometimes useful as an alternative to the erect abdominal radiograph in patients who are unfit to sit or stand.

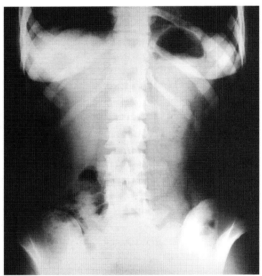

FIG 2—Erect abdominal radiograph showing free air under both hemidiaphragms (pneumoperitoneum).

Causes of air-fluid levels on erect abdominal radiograph

Ileus
Obstruction
Gastroenteritis
Ischaemia
Hypokalaemia or uraemia
Normal (<2·5 cm in length)

Radiological assessment of supine abdominal radiograph

Check the adequacy and quality of the radiograph

The radiograph should include the area from the diaphragm to the hernial orifices. Laterally the proportional line should be evident.

Summary for checking bones

Ribs
Lumbar vertebrae and appendages (especially transverse processes)
Sacrum
Pelvis:
　Iliac crest
　Acetabula
　Pubis
Femoral head and neck

Check alignment of bones

Examination of the lumbar spine will be covered in the article on the thoracolumbar spine.

Check bone margins and density

The abdominal radiograph shows many portions of the skeleton that can be injured after blunt or penetrating trauma. The lower ribs and lumbar transverse processes must be examined carefully. If fractures of these bones are seen consider associated soft tissue injury to the liver, spleen, or kidney.

Check the cartilage and joints
See the chapter on the pelvis for details.

Check soft tissues
Bowel gas pattern—Gas and faecal matter in the gastrointestinal tract delineate the distribution of the bowel as well as indirectly identify intra-abdominal organs. Almost all patients in distress with abdominal pain swallow air, which rapidly passes through the bowel (fig 1). The stomach is often partly filled with air and it can be located by the characteristic appearance of the gastric rugae. A small amount of gas is often seen in the duodenal bulb and in various parts of normal small bowel, which does not exceed 2·5 cm in diameter. The valvulae conniventes appear relatively thick. The amount of gas in the colon is extremely variable.

Assessing cartilage and joints

Pubic symphysis—Widening or overlapping of bone
Sacroiliac joint—Widening or overlapping of bone, defects in cortical surface
Acetabulum—Check for fractures

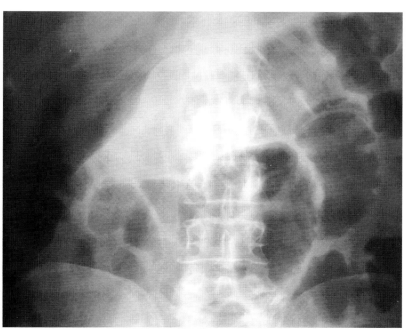

FIG 3—Perforated duodenal ulcer with a large amount of free air overlying the liver.

Free air and air in biliary tree or portal vein—Pneumoperitoneum is a result of perforation of a viscus, unless the patient has recently had a laparotomy. The commonest cause is perforated peptic ulcer, but free air is evident in only 70-80% of such cases (figs 2 and 3). In a supine radiograph intraperitoneal air collects under the inferior surface of the liver or hepatorenal recess (Morison's pouch). Small triangular collections of air may also be evident between adjacent loops of bowel. Larger collections rise to lie under the central tendon of the diaphragm (capula sign) or outline the falciform ligament. Visibility of both sides of the bowel wall (Rigler's sign; fig 4) is important but may be misleading when two loops of air filled bowel are in apposition. Occasionally air is seen outlining the gall bladder or urinary bladder in diabetic patients with emphysematous infections.

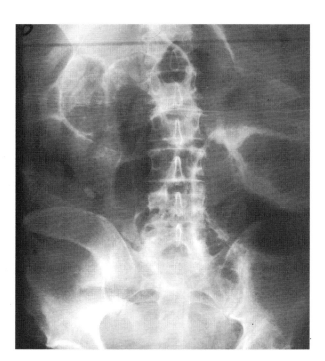

FIG 4—Pneumoperitoneum as shown by Rigler's sign—both sides of the bowel wall can be seen . There are multiple dilated small bowel loops and gall stones in the gall bladder.

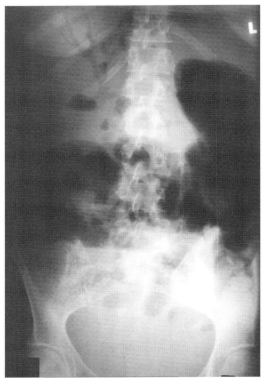

FIG 5—Air in biliary tree from previous endoscopic sphincterotomy. The patient has also had a bowel resection for carcinoma—note surgical sutures to the right of L4/5 disc space. Only a little gas is seen in the pelvis where there is increased soft tissue density because of localised ascites.

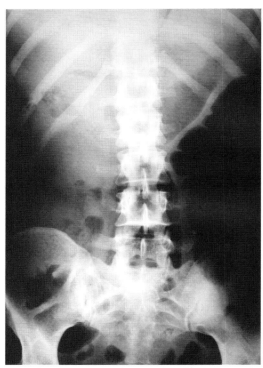

FIG 6—Right paracolic abscess showing increased density in the right flank and displacement of the colonic gas medially. A few locules of extraluminal gas are seen within the abscess cavity, overlying the right 11th rib.

Check size of organs

Identification of the organs within the abdomen depends on knowledge of their anatomical position, helped by the tissue-fat interfaces and the adjacent bowel, which contains gas, fluid, and food residue. The soft tissue density of the liver, spleen, and kidneys can usually be seen in this view (fig 1).

The size and shape of the liver is extremely variable and its posterior edge can extend down to the region of the iliac crest (Riedel's lobe). With severe hepatomegaly the hepatic flexure, transverse colon, or stomach is usually displaced with a raised right hemidiaphragm. The pancreas cannot be seen in plain abdominal films unless it is calcified.

Check fat and soft tissue interfaces

The borders of the kidneys, psoas muscles, bladder, and properitoneal line can usually be seen in an abdominal radiograph because of the interface between these structures and the surrounding retroperitoneal fat (fig 1). Remember, however, that their visibility and appearance are not consistent. The right psoas outline is not seen in a fifth of the normal population.

The visibility of the psoas shadow also depends on overlying normal structures such as bowel contents, as well as on pathological conditions (retroperitoneal haemorrhage in kidney trauma, fractures of the vertebral spinous processes, or psoas haematoma). Fluid within the paracolic gutter causes displacement of the colon medially, increasing the width of the soft tissue density between the properitoneal line and the intraluminal colonic contents (fig 6).

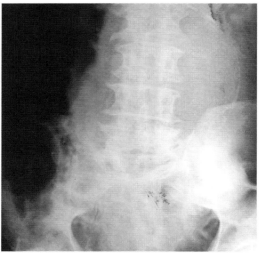

FIG 7—Soft tissue density mass in mid-abdomen with curvilinear calcification This represents large abdominal aortic aneurysm.

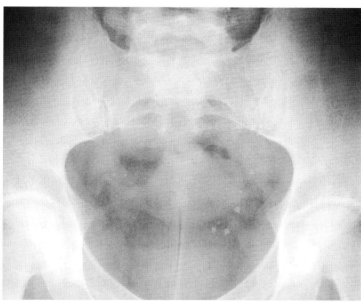

FIG 8—Typical pelvic phleboliths. Note apparent soft tissue mass in the pelvis due to the uterus. The uterus can be seen because of surrounding pelvic fat.

Check for abnormal calcification

The commonest calcified structures seen in the abdominal radiograph are pelvic phleboliths due to pelvic vein thrombosis and lymph nodes. About 85% of renal stones are radio-opaque, compared with only 15% of gall stones. Renal stones can be suspected by the presence of a stone overlying the renal outline or ureter (fig 9). Occasionally punctate pancreatic calcification is seen in patients with chronic pancreatitis.

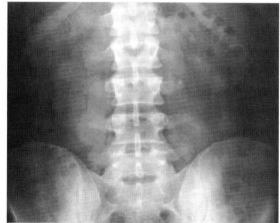

FIG 9—A small ureteric calculus is projected over the left L3 transverse process.

Catches to avoid

The properitoneal line adjacent to the lateral margin of the liver can be mistaken for a pneumoperitoneum in a left lateral decubitus view. Air in the biliary tree can be due to previous sphincterotomy or surgery (fig 5). Pelvic phleboliths can often be differentiated from distal ureteric stones by their characteristic appearance; they are round with a radio-opaque halo surrounding a small central lucent nidus.

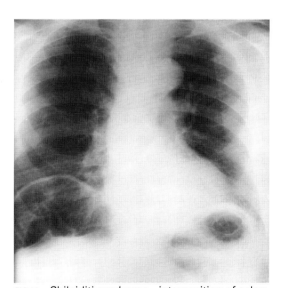

FIG 10—Chilaiditi syndrome—interposition of colon between liver and diaphragm. Air is seen under the right hemidiaphragm but bowel markings are evident.

Conditions simulating air under the diaphragm

Chilaiditi syndrome (fig 10)—
Interposition of hepatic flexure between liver and diaphragm
Subphrenic abscess
Subdiaphragmatic fat
Basal curvilinear atelectasis

Radiographic signs of trauma

Radiographic signs of splenic injury

Normal abdominal radiograph

Raised left hemidiaphragm ⎫
Left pleural effusion ⎬ Classic triad
Left basal atelectasis ⎭

Left lower rib fracture

Left upper quadrant mass and medial displacement of gastric air bubble or inferomedial displacement of splenic flexure

Splenic enlargement—usually with subcapsular haemorrhage

Haemoperitoneum—see text

Splenic injury cannot be excluded by a normal abdominal or chest radiograph

Death after blunt abdominal trauma is usually due to massive splenic or hepatic haemorrhage—in such patients laparotomy should not be delayed

Signs of retroperitoneal haemorrhage

Bulging of lateral margin of psoas shadow (bleeding confined by muscle fascia)
Obliteration of psoas shadow (free blood)
Concave lumber scoliosis
Loss of definition of renal outline
Ipsilateral fractures of lower ribs or lumbar transverse processes

Blunt injuries

Clinical examination is notoriously difficult, and although an abdominal radiograph can be taken as a first line investigation, often other imaging methods such as ultrasonography and computed tomography are needed to assess patients with multiple injuries who are haemodynamically stable and therefore do not require urgent laparotomy.

Splenic injury—Splenic rupture is the most common serious injury associated with blunt trauma in the upper abdomen. It may result in subcapsular haemorrhage with an intact capsule or capsular disruption, which is evident by intraperitoneal bleeding and haemorrhagic shock. Blood usually accumulates in the left paracolic gutter, producing increased soft tissue density between the descending colon and the properitoneal line. A raised left hemidiaphragm should always be considered suspicious, although this can occur normally.

Hepatic injury should be suspected in patients with a fracture of the right lower rib. Concomitant splenic injury is reported in up to a quarter of cases. A fifth show no signs or symptoms because the rupture is confined by the capsule.

Intestinal injury—The small and large intestine are rarely damaged on their own. Most patients have other more obvious injuries. Rupture of the third part of duodenum is the most common site, with signs of retroperitoneal haemorrhage or air surrounding the right kidney.

Penetrating injuries

Penetrating injuries resulting from high energy transfer are often so severe that the patient's condition will not allow formal radiographic studies. In haemodynamically stable patients, abdominal radiography is valuable for localising foreign bodies and assessing associated skeletal or soft tissue damage.

Abdominal gunshot wounds are a special problem in preoperative evaluation. Renal function often needs to be assessed urgently to exclude serious renal vascular damage. This can be done by taking an abdominal radiograph five minutes after giving intravenous iodinated contrast media.

Radiographic signs of the acute abdomen

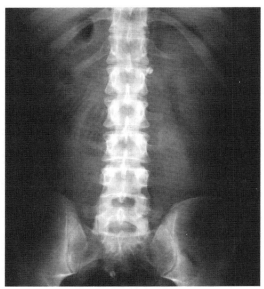

FIG 11—Isolated, dilated loop of duodenum in a patient with acute pancreatitis (sentinel loop sign).

Ileus

The visibility of distended loops of bowel depends on the air and fluid content. Ileus can be generalised or localised to a segment of bowel due to a focal inflammatory process such as appendicitis, cholecystitis, or pancreatitis. This gives rise to the sentinal loop sign.

Mechanical obstruction

Mechanical obstruction can be partial or complete, with the distribution of distension depending on the site of obstruction.

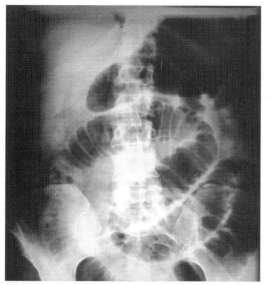

FIG 12—Complete small bowel obstruction due to surgical adhesions. The stomach and proximal small bowel are air filled and dilated. No gas is seen in the large bowel.

Small bowel obstruction—Dilated small bowel loops are usually evident three to five hours after the onset of complete obstruction (fig 12). They are identified by their central distribution, the presence of close valvulae conniventes that extend across the entire diameter of the bowel, and the absence of faeces. As small bowel obstruction progresses the distal bowel collapses and the colon becomes void of air. If the gut is largely fluid filled small amounts of air collect in the recesses between the valvulae conniventes, producing a chain of small radiolucent bubbles referred to as the string of pearl sign. Distended loops that are almost completely filled with fluid can be misinterpreted as ascites.

Large bowel obstruction—Dilated colon is identified by its peripheral distribution, haustral sacculations (which are thick and extend only a short distance into the gas filled lumen), and faecal content (fig 13). The distribution of bowel gas and the risk of perforation depend on the competency of the ileocaecal valve. With a competent valve the caecum is most likely to perforate as it is the most compliant region of the large bowel and distends more rapidly and to a greater degree than the remaining colon. With an incompetent ileocaecal valve, the caecum is decompressed by air passing into the small bowel. If the obstruction is complete and long standing, the gastrointestinal tract will eventually decompensate and become atonic as in ileus.

Pseudo-obstruction mimics obstruction clinically and radiologically but no obstructing lesion is found (fig 14). There is diffuse dilatation of the small and large bowel, often with prominent gastric distension. Barium enema or flexible sigmoidoscopy are often needed to differentiate pseudo-obstruction from organic obstruction.

Causes of small bowel obstruction

Adhesions due to previous surgery (75%)

Strangulated hernias (10%)

Appendix abscess

Gall stone ileus (2%— commoner in women, up to 25% in elderly patients)

Crohn's disease

Tumour

Intussusception

Volvulus

Commonest causes of large bowel obstruction

Carcinoma (commonly sigmoid or rectosigmoid)

Diverticular disease

Volvulus (10%)

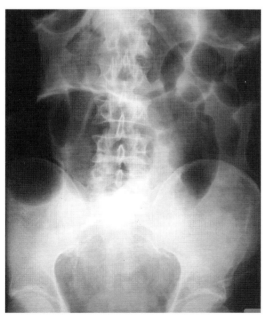

FIG 13—Large bowel obstruction due to obstructing carcinoma in the descending colon. The large bowel is dilated to the level of obstruction. No air is seen distal to this in the sigmoid colon or rectum.

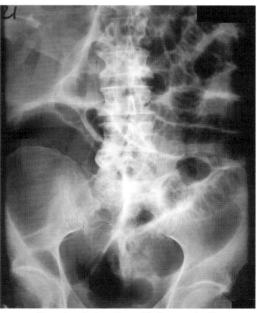

FIG 14—Pseudo-obstruction. Air is seen in the rectum and throughout the dilated small and large bowel. The caecum is massively distended to 15 cm and at a high risk of perforation. No organic lesion was found.

Volvulus—Volvulus causes closed obstruction of loops, resulting in both proximal and distal portions of a loop of bowel being completely occluded. It occurs where the mesentery of the gut is longest, the most common sites being the sigmoid colon and caecum. Volvulus of the transverse colon or duodenum is rare.

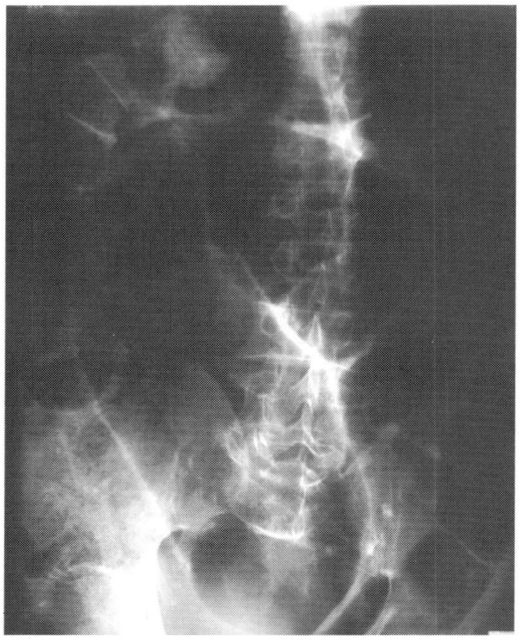

In sigmoid volvulus there is classically a greatly dilated loop of colon, devoid of haustra, arising from the left side of the pelvis and projecting obliquely upwards to the right side of the abdomen (fig 15). The volvulus overlies the distended descending colon (left flank overlap sign) and inferior border of liver (liver overlap sign). The central stripe is characteristic and is produced by the adjacent walls of the upper and lower limb of the volvulus.

Even with severe distension in caecal volvulus two haustral markings are usually identifiable. The left side of the colon is collapsed, but small bowel dilatation is often clearly seen. In half of patients with caecal volvulus the caecal pole inverts to lie in the left upper quadrant. In this orientation the wall of the dilated caecum is often kidney shaped. In the other half the twist is in the axial plane (without inversion) with the caecum remaining in the right lower quadrant.

Gall stone ileus—Gall stone ileus is the term given to mechanical obstruction caused by a gall stone that has passed into the gastrointestinal tract by eroding through the inflamed gall bladder wall (fig 16). The usual site of impaction is the pelvic or terminal ileum. Specific radiological signs are present in only 40%. These include gas in the biliary tree (30%), partial or complete small bowel obstruction (50%), and visible ectopic gall stone (35%).

Intussusception is most common in children under the age of 2 years and is often due to lymphoid hyperplasia in the terminal ileum. Small bowel obstruction is seen in the abdominal radiograph possibly with a soft tissue mass surrounded by a crescent of air (fig 17).

FIG 15—Classic appearance of sigmoid volvulus. The volvulus appears as a dilated, folded loop of bowel originating from the left side of the pelvis with a coffee bean configuration.

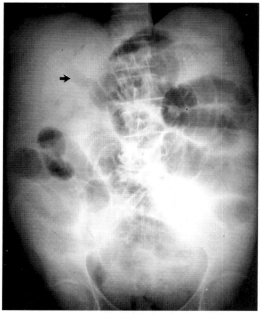

FIG 16—Gall stone ileus showing multiple, dilated, air filled loops of small bowel and gas in the biliary tree (arrow). No air is seen in the large bowel, suggesting small bowel obstruction. The gall stone is often non-opaque or obscured and therefore not identified, as in this case.

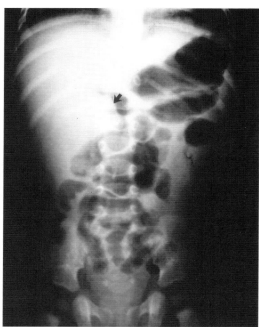

FIG 17—Intussusception in an infant. There are multiple dilated, air filled loops of bowel. The head of the ileocaecal intussusceptus can be seen in the region of the transverse colon, overlying the spine (arrow).

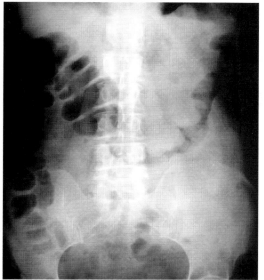

FIG 18—Ischaemic colitis of the splenic flexure with narrowing and severe submucosal haemorrhage in the distal transverse colon (thumb printing).

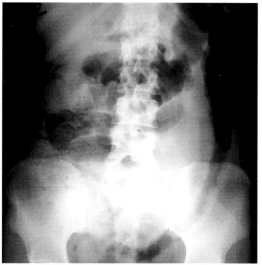

FIG 19—Acute ulcerative colitis showing oedematous left colon, which is narrowed and shortened. A cut off is seen in the transverse colon with faecal loading of the right colon due to functional obstruction.

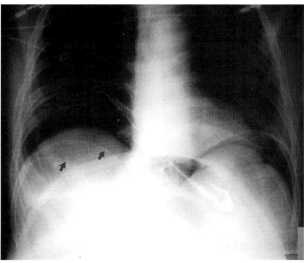

FIG 20—Erect chest radiograph showing a large pneumoperitoneum with air under both diaphragms. The right hemidiaphragm is raised. Dilated air filled loops of bowel are projected over the liver (arrows)—both sides of the bowel wall can be seen (Rigler's sign).

Bowel ischaemia

The early radiological features of bowel ischaemia mimic mechanical obstruction but as the vascular occlusion progresses the bowel wall becomes oedematous and necrotic. This is seen as severe thickening of the bowel wall associated with obstruction.

Ischaemic colitis most commonly affects the splenic flexure and descending colon, with submucosal haemorrhage causing thickening of the colonic wall. These changes are seen as thumb printing (fig 18). Functional obstruction with dilatation of the proximal colon is commonly seen. As the ischaemia progresses linear gas may be identified in the bowel wall, indicating necrosis. Free gas indicates perforation, and the presence of gas in the portal vein is a serious prognostic sign.

Acute inflammatory colitis

The distribution of faecal material is a good indicator of the extent of inflammation of the bowel wall. In ulcerative colitis there is usually a sharp cut off from normal bowel, which is identified by the distal limit of the faecal residue (fig 19). With extensive mucosal ulceration small normal mucosal islands are left (pseudopolyps), which can be seen in the plain film.

Occasionally a gasless colon is seen in a patient with severe ulcerative colitis. When the transverse colonic diameter exceeds 5·5 cm megacolon should be diagnosed, and when this is associated with fever, tachycardia, leucocytosis, and pain toxic megacolon exists. Perforation and peritonitis are common sequelae (fig 20).

Acute pancreatitis

In most patients no plain film abnormality is identified (fig 11). The signs most frequently seen, however, are a dilated duodenal sentinal loop, loss of the left psoas margin, signs of gastric outlet obstruction, and left sided pleural effusion. These features are non-specific.

Summary

Diagnostic quality

Alignment of bones

Bone margins and density

Cartilage and joints

Soft tissues
Bowel gas pattern
Pneumoperitoneum
Air in the biliary tree or portal vein
Size of organs
Fat-tissue interfaces
Abnormal calcification

PELVIS

P A Driscoll, R Ross, D A Nicholson

> It is possible for the non-specialist to interpret pelvic radiographs accurately

This chapter describes a system by which non-specialists can interpret pelvic radiographs. It requires an awareness of the basic anatomy of the region and an understanding of the possible mechanisms of injury. These two aspects will be discussed first.

Important anatomical considerations

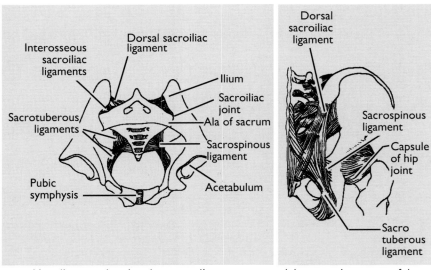

FIG 1—Line diagram showing the strong ligaments around the posterior aspect of the pelvis. Left: anterior view. Right: posterior view.

Adult

The pelvis is composed of three bones (the sacrum and the two innominate bones) held together by several extremely strong ligaments. These are crucial for maintaining pelvic stability.

A large complex of ligaments covers the interior and exterior surface of the posterior aspect of the pelvis (fig 1). In addition, there are two ligaments that originate from the side and back of the sacrum and insert into the ischial spine and ischial tuberosity.

Branches of the internal iliac vessels and lumbosacral nerve plexus are closely aligned to the sacrotuberous, sacrospinous, and anterior sacroiliac ligaments and the underlying sacroiliac joint (fig 2).

The pubic symphysis is a fibrocartilagenous joint which is supported by ligaments and adds only a little to the overall stability of the pelvis. However, the urethra and bladder lie close to the pubic symphysis and are consequently damaged in a fifth of cases when this area is disrupted.

The three bones of the pelvis can separate only when the ligaments are torn. When this happens the nerves and vessels running close to them will also be damaged. The bleeding is usually venous and extraperitoneal and can be life threatening. If bones fracture but the ligaments remain intact, a tamponade effect can be achieved and the degree of haemorrhage limited.

Developmental

Epiphyseal lines may be misinterpreted as fractures because the apophyses of the ischial tuberosity, lesser trochanter, and iliac crest do not unite until the end of the late teens.

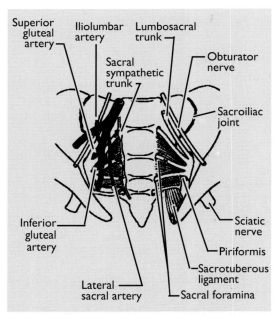

FIG 2—Line diagram showing close relation of internal iliac vessels, ligaments, and sacroiliac joint.

Mechanism of injury

Patterns of force leading to pelvic damage
Anteroposterior compression
Lateral compression
Vertical shear
Complex (combination) pattern

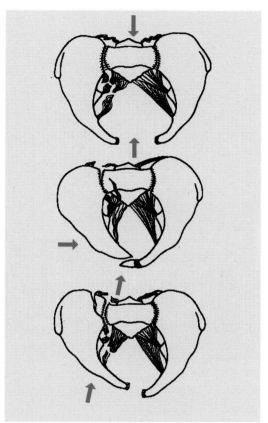

FIG 3—Forces on the pelvis. From top to bottom: anteroposterior compression, lateral compression, and vertical shear

There are four patterns of force leading to pelvic damage (fig 3).

Anteroposterior compression

Anteroposterior compression causes one or both sides of the pelvis to open up like a book, with the spine of the "book" running down the sacrum. A diffuse force will disrupt the pubic symphysis, while a more direct force fractures the pubic rami in a vertical plane. Occasionally a combination occurs.

For the pubic bones to separate by over 2·5 cm, one or both of the ligaments associated with the sacroiliac joints have to be torn. If the sacroiliac ligaments are stronger than their bony insertion an avulsion fracture of the ilium will be produced.

An anteroposterior force can also push the flexed femur backwards so that the femoral head impacts and fractures the posterior margin of the acetabular rim.

Lateral compression

Lateral compression produces a compression fracture of the ala of the sacrum, a horizontal fracture through the ipsilateral pubic symphysis, and a momentary medial displacement of the hemipelvis. The extent of this movement depends on the amount of force and the point of impact.

A lateral compression force can also impinge on the upper femur causing central dislocation of the hip (see later).

Vertical shear force

This forces the hemipelvis upwards and towards the midline and can tear all the sacroiliac ligaments on the affected side as well as the ligaments of the pubic symphysis. Because of the ligamental damage a vertical shearing injury is associated with severe pelvic instability and vascular damage.

Complex pattern

In less than a quarter of cases, the pelvis is subjected to two or more of the forces mentioned above. A combination of injuries results in a complex radiological picture. Nevertheless, the radiograph can usually still be interpreted by using the principles mentioned in this chapter.

Interpretation of the anteroposterior radiograph

Types of pelvic views
Routine
Anteroposterior projection
Special
Inlet and outlet views
Oblique views (Judet) of the acetabulum

ABCs system of radiographic interpretation
Alignment
Bones
Cartilage and joints
Soft tissues

In 94% of cases a correct diagnoses can be made from only an anteroposterior radiograph of the pelvis.

A disciplined approach is important when interpreting pelvic radiographs. Once the adequacy of the film has been determined, we recommend using the ABCs system.

Check the adequacy and quality of the film

Ensure that the whole of the pelvis can be seen, including the iliac crests, both hips, and the femurs distal to the lesser trochanters. The adequacy of the penetration should also be assessed. Pelvic rotation is determined by lining up the symphysis pubis with the midline of the sacrum.

Alignment

The pelvis encloses three circles. One is created by the pelvic brim and the other two by the obturator foramina (fig 4).

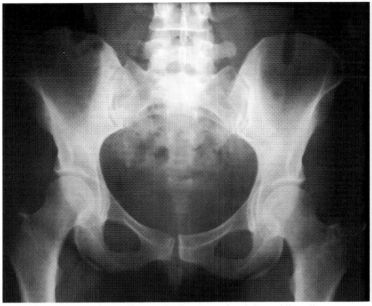

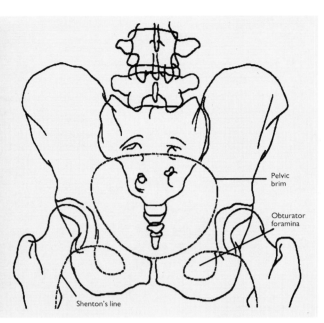

FIG 4—Anteroposterior radiograph of a normal pelvis and line diagram with the three circles and Shenton's line traced out.

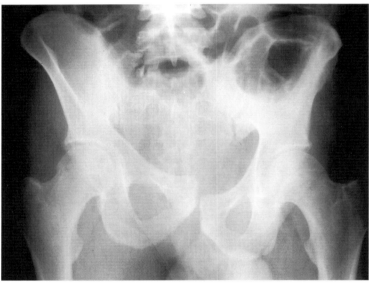

FIG 5—Disruption of the pelvic brim due to a vertical shear injury on the right side. There is also disruption of the sacroiliac joint—the upper surface of the sacrum on the right has fractured and lies immediately below the transverse process of L5 (enlargement).

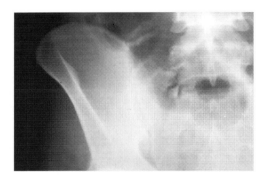

Pelvic brim—Trace around the rim of the large circle. Normally this has a smooth edge which is not disrupted by the sacroiliac joint or pubic symphysis unless the patient is very old. Once a fracture or diastasis is found, check for a second disruption in the circle (fig 5). As the pelvis is not completely rigid, this disruption may take the form of a minimal diastasis, which can be difficult to see.

> The pelvic brim cannot be disrupted in only one place.

Avulsion fractures due to ligamental strain have the same effect as a rupture of the corresponding ligament. They are therefore important to detect in the plain radiograph. For example, avulsion of the ischial spine indicates that there has been an anteroposterior compression force sufficient to compromise the sacroiliac ligament.

Obturator foramina—The inner margins of both obturator foramina should then be inspected in the same way as the pelvic brim. Again these are rarely broken in only one place. Complete the examination of the foramina by tracing along their superior border to the inferior surface of the neck of the femur. This is known as Shenton's line. Disruption of this normally smooth line indicates that the femoral neck is broken (fig 6).

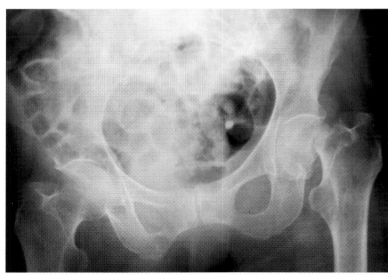

FIG 6—Anteroposterior showing disruption of Shenton's line due to a left femoral neck fracture.

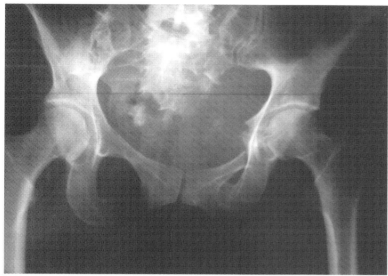

FIG 7—Anteroposterior radiograph showing disruption of lines around the acetabulum due to a central dislocation of the left hip. The soft tissue shadow associated with the obturator internus muscle is absent on the left but present on the right.

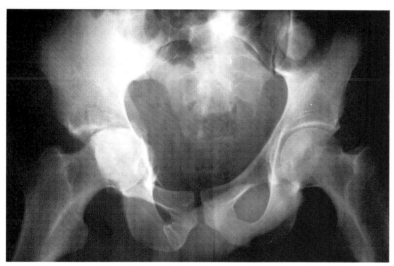

FIG 8—Anteroposterior radiograph showing several abnormalities after lateral compression injury. The pelvic brim on the right is disrupted because of fracture of the superior and inferior pubic rami. The right iliopectineal and ilioischial line is also disrupted because of a central dislocation of the hip and a sacral fracture has disrupted the right upper sacral foramina (enlargement).

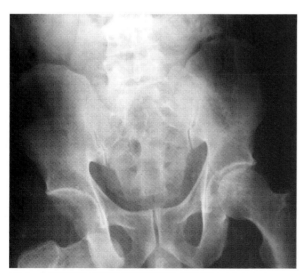

FIG 9—Anteroposterior radiograph showing a fracture of the posterior aspect of the left acetabulum and dislocation of the right hip.

Bones

Examine the outer edges of the pelvis and its bony structure for evidence of fractures. These may present as areas of increased density, lucency, or alteration of internal trabecular pattern. Fractures away from the three bony circles can occur in isolation.

Start the examination at the pubic symphysis and progress to either the right or the left. To prevent getting lost in all the radio-opaque lines of the acetabular fossa concentrate, from lateral to medial, on the posterior and anterior joint margin, the ilioischial line (posterior column), and the iliopectineal line (anterior column) and finish with the tear drop sign (acetabular floor) (fig 7 and hip chapter fig 1).

Next examine the anterior inferior iliac spine and progress to the anterior superior iliac spine and over the iliac crest to the sacrum. The sacrum should also be examined for symmetry of its foramina (fig 8). A break in the smooth border of a sacral foramina may be the only indicator of a lateral crush fracture.

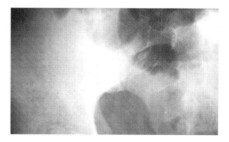

The contralateral ilium, acetabulum, rami, and pubis are then examined. Finally the femoral heads and lumbar vertebrae are inspected. The cortical margins, trabecular pattern, and bone density should be assessed. Isolated fractures away from the pelvic rim or obturator foramina can occur.

Cartilage and joints

Pubic symphysis—Check for either widening or overlapping of bone. Such an injury will be associated with disruption elsewhere in the pelvic brim.

Sacroiliac joints—The right and left sides must be checked for widening, defects in the cortical surface, overlapping of bone, and lack of congruity of the joint margin.

Acetabulum—Fractures can be detected by tracing over the cortical margins. Posterior and anterior acetabular rim fractures can be easily missed because they are covered by the shadow of the femoral head. Look for isolated bone fragments lying behind the femoral head (fig 9).

The commonest fracture to the acetabulum is in the posterior rim after a posterior dislocation of the hip. Occasionally a lateral force produces a central dislocation by pushing the femoral head through the floor of the acetabulum. However, this may have sprung back by the time the radiograph is taken, leaving only subtle soft tissue signs. Fractures of the anterior rim and column are rare.

Soft tissue—internal and external

Check for soft tissue shadowing both inside and outside the pelvis because haematoma and tissue oedema can produce swellings which are visible on the anteroposterior radiograph.

Normally the obturator internus muscle is seen on both sides of the pelvis as a dark grey line, which is due to the muscle or fat plane (fig 7). Loss of this line indicates extraperitoneal haemorrhage or soft tissue oedema. Conversely, intraperitoneal haemorrhage can displace the line.

Special views

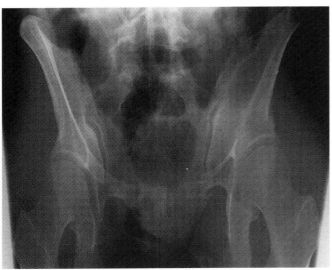

Inlet and outlet views

Inlet and outlet views should ideally be requested if there is clinical or radiological evidence of a pelvic fracture.

An inlet view looks down the lumen of the true pelvis. It is better than the anteroposterior view for showing the orientation of fractures of the pubic rami. Outlet views are used to detect the degree of vertical displacement of the fracture fragments.

FIG 10—Inlet view of pelvis showing a fracture of the left superior and inferior rami.

Inlet and outlet views should be requested only after consultation with a specialist and if the patient's clinical state is good enough to tolerate further investigation

Oblique (Judet) views

These are used to define acetabular fracture patterns. If a fracture or abnormality of the acetabulum is suspected computed tomography will usually be necessary once the patient has been adequately resuscitated and stabilised.

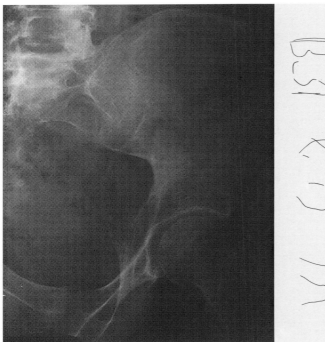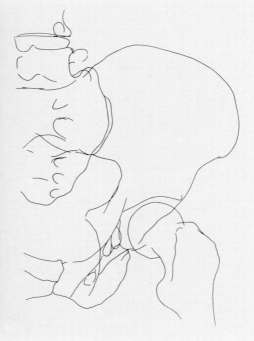

FIG 11—Judet view and line diagram of a normal left hip.

Catches to avoid

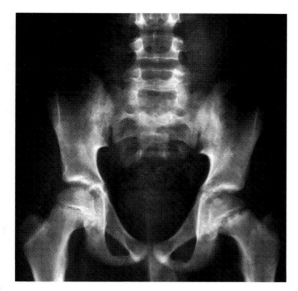

Make sure the radiograph is adequate. Commonly part of the iliac crest is missing or the film is poorly penetrated so that fractures cannot be seen. A rotated film causes asymmetry of the bony circles and the sacroiliac joints.

FIG 12—Anteroposterior radiograph of a child's pelvis. Notice the epiphyseal lines and the bilateral ischiopubic knobs. The left capital epiphysis has slipped slightly compared with the right.

Failing to trace around the bony edges, especially the iliac crests and sacral foramina, will lead to fractures being missed.

Epiphyseal lines may be misinterpreted as fractures. Remember that the Y-shaped (triradiate) cartilage separating the pubis, ischium, and ilium in the acetabular floor does not fuse until puberty. Accessory ossification centres (in particular the one in the posterior acetabulum) may also be mistaken for fractures. However, apophyses are usually bilateral, have a sclerotic margin, and are not associated with overlying soft tissue signs.

Summary

Adequacy and quality
Ensure that the whole of the pelvis is visible

Alignment
Assess the borders of the three circles—namely, the pelvic brim and the two obturator foramina

Bones
Check each of the following systematically:

Pubis	Sacrum
Acetabulum	Femoral heads
Iliac crest	Lumbar vertebrae

Cartilage and joints
Check the pubic symphysis
Check the sacroiliac joints
Check the acetabulum

Soft tissues
Check the disruption of fat planes inside the pelvis
Check for soft tissue shadows outside the pelvis

SKULL

D A Nicholson, P A Driscoll, D W Hodgkinson, W St C Forbes

> Patients with a skull fracture or other serious head injury should be admitted to hospital

Many thousands of skull radiographs are requested each year by doctors treating patients with head injuries. Unfortunately, most are taken when direct consultation with a radiologist is not possible. This chapter describes an effective system by which non-radiologists can analyse skull radiographs. To do this it is important to consider certain anatomical points so that normal features can be recognised.

Important anatomical considerations

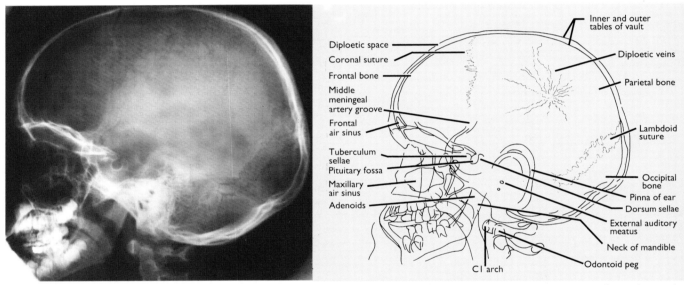

FIG 1—Normal lateral skull radiograph and line diagram showing typical appearances of lambdoid and coronal sutures. Several vascular markings are seen, including a stellate venous lake in the parietal bone and normal soft tissue adenoids.

Causes of intracranial calcification

Normal
  Pineal gland
  Choroid plexuses
  Dural (commonly falx)
  Vascular (carotid arteries)
  Basal ganglia

Abnormal
  Tumours (craniopharyngioma,
    meningioma, glioma, etc)
  Arteriovenous malformation (15%)
  Aneurysms (1%)
  Vault or sinus osteoma

Adults

The shape of the skull varies among races and these variations can be incorrectly interpreted as abnormalities—for example, natives from the Middle East classically have a short high broad vault with parietal bossing and flattening of the occiput.

The cranium can be divided into the vault (calvaria) and the skull base. The calvaria is divided into inner and outer tables by the intervening diploetic space, and the skull base is divided into anterior, middle, and posterior fossae. Straight lines can be caused by vascular markings from meningeal vascular grooves, venous diploetic channels, and occasionally subcutaneous or periosteal vessels. These lines can be difficult to distinguish from fractures.

The pineal gland, which lies at the apex of the tentorium, may become calcified and up to 1 cm in diameter without any abnormality. Normal calcification can also be identified in various other structures. Hyperostosis frontalis interna is irregular, corrugated calcification (more common in women) of the inner table of the frontal bone, which in most patients is an incidental finding.

Children

There are several fundamental differences between the skulls of adults and children. At birth the calvaria is relatively large compared with the face and base of skull (fig 2). Ectopic ossification centres are often seen along the sutures, giving rise to intrasutural (wormian) bones. These anomalous bones are often multiple and symmetrical and are most commonly found along the lambdoid and sagittal sutures; although they usually do not indicate disease, they can be associated with congenital bone abnormalities.

> Brain injury can occur without skull vault fracture and vice versa

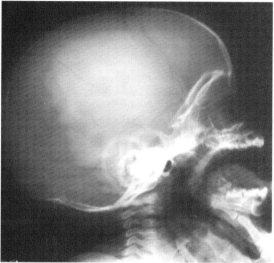

FIG 2—Simple linear parietal fracture in infant. Note the sheno-occipital synchondrosis (see enlargement).

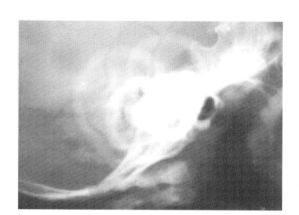

As the skull grows from birth the bones thicken, though not uniformly. The squamous temporal, frontal, and occipital bones remain at a lower density and therefore appear relatively translucent (fig 1). The bones are incompletely mineralised and separated by radiolucent sutures and fontanelles.

The great sutures (sagittal, coronal, lambdoid) persist into adult life. At birth they can measure up to 1 cm, but by 3 years the suture width has reduced to 2 mm. The frontal bone is divided in two by the frontal or metopic suture, which usually fuses by the age of 3 years. Vascular markings on the inner table are evident from 2 to 3 years onwards.

Criteria for skull radiography after recent head injury

- Loss of consciousness or amnesia at any time
- Neurological symptoms and signs
- Leak of bloody cerebrospinal fluid from nose or ear
- Suspected penetrating injury or foreign body
- Tense fontanelle, scalp bruising, or laceration (to bone or >5 cm long), falls from height (>60 cm or on to hard surface in under 5 year olds)
- People who live alone or in a domestic situation that precludes proper surveillance
- Presence of other trauma that might imply a strong force of impact
- Presence of other conditions—for example, stroke, epileptic seizure, mental handicap—that might preclude proper examination
- People with alcoholic intoxication

Types of view

Standard radiographic projections

Lateral—right or left according to side of injury

Anteroposterior

Half-axial (Towne's)

Radiological investigations should be carried out after completing the ABCs of trauma resuscitation. This will include stabilisation of a patient's neck until a cervical injury has been ruled out clinically and radiologically.

There are three standard skull projections. The half axial view is contraindicated in patients with suspected cervical injury. In addition, it is not advisable to attempt the complete series on patients who are restless or uncooperative. Patients with serious head injuries should have computed tomography rather than skull radiography.

Assessment of lateral skull radiograph

The lateral view (fig 1) is the most important projection.

> Important management decisions depend on detecting or excluding fractures. When present fractures can help determine possible outcome

Check adequacy and alignment

Start by establishing the adequacy of the radiograph, which includes the exposure (film blackening), the centring of the radiograph, and rotation. The anterior clinoid processes and posterior margins of the mandible should be superimposed. Non-diagnostic radiographs should be repeated provided that the patient's condition permits.

Bone margins and density

Check the sellae—From the tuberculum sellae trace the cortical margin of the pituitary fossa posteriorly to the dorsum sellae. Check the radiograph for rotation if a double floor is seen. Looking at the sella (sphenoid fossa) can help distinguish between head injury and other causes of impaired consciousness such as longstanding raised intracranial pressure or pressure erosion or truncation from a midline brain tumour. The floor (lamina dura) should have a single margin that can be traced to the dorsum sellae (fig 1). The commonest cause of erosion is raised intracranial pressure (which needs to be present for at least four weeks), but in elderly patients you should consider osteoporosis causing a blurred cortex. There is a wide variation in both normal and pathological entities, but nevertheless the shape of the sellae should also be noted.

Normal size of pituitary fossa

Height 6·5-11 mm
Length 9-16 mm
Breadth 9-19 mm

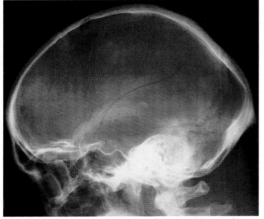

FIG 3—Simple linear fracture of parietal bone. Note the pineal calcification.

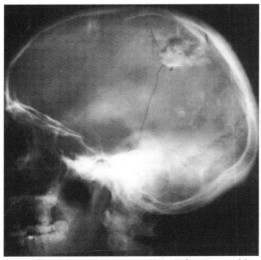

FIG 4—Complicated depressed vault fracture, with linear component extending into the parietal bone. Soft tissue abnormality from dirt is seen behind the fracture.

Check the calvaria and skull base for fractures—Continue from the dorsum sellae to the occipital bone, which can be difficult to see because of the density of the overlying petrous bone. Over the vault look for defects of the inner and outer tables. Next assess the anterior fossa floor followed by the en-face portions of the frontal, parietal, and occipital bones.

Skull fractures can be of three types: linear (fig 3), depressed, and stellate. Linear fractures are the most common and are usually uncomplicated. Depressed fractures can indicate that the brain substance is in direct communication with the outside—that is, an open injury. An area of double density, representing the overlapping bone, will be found opposite a translucent area (fig 4). Tangential views are useful to assess the degree of depression, but computed tomography is now routinely performed when this is suspected. If the bone fragment is depressed more than 0·5 cm surgery is needed to raise it. Stellate lesions are generally easier to detect, with the central point usually being the site of a sharp impact. Tangential views should be taken as some depression can coexist.

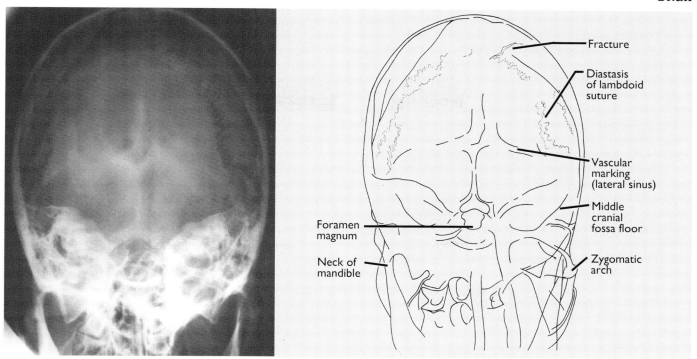

FIG 5—Towne's projection showing diastasis of right lambdoid suture with an associated short linear fracture of parietal bone.

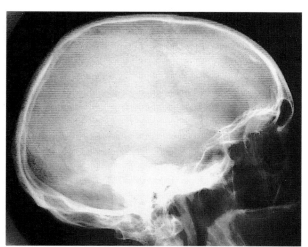

FIG 6—Fracture through C1 with displacement. Note the soft tissue swelling.

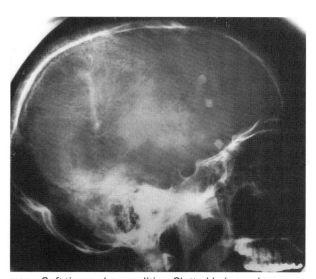

FIG 7—Soft tissue abnormalities. Clotted hair causing linear artefact posteriorly and multiple square fragments of glass are seen anteriorly.

Cartilage and joints

Check the sutures—The upper limit of normal for width of suture depends on the patient's age. Occasionally fractures occur along the line of a suture, causing diastasis (fig 5). With raised intracranial pressure widening of sutures is seen a few days after injury in children, but it is rare in adults.

Check the craniocervical region—The upper cervical spine is commonly overlooked on the skull radiograph but it may show valuable signs indicating associated neck injury (fig 6). In children the adenoids form a large soft tissue mass in the postnasal space (fig 1). In adults widening of this area suggests haemorrhage and associated cervical spine injury. Malalignment at the craniocervical junction can be highly important in major acute head injury but initially it may be masked by other changes. The normal distance from the posteroinferior aspect of C1 to the anterior aspect of the odontoid peg is <3 mm in adults and < 5 mm in children.

Soft tissues

Finally, examine the soft tissues for foreign bodies or artefacts with a bright light. Hair preparations and plaits or beads in the hair can cause discrepancies in overall density. Opaque foreign bodies may be penetrating missiles or bony fragments (fig 7). Two views at right angles to each other are needed to ascertain their position (intracranial or superficial). If penetration is suspected computed tomography is indicated.

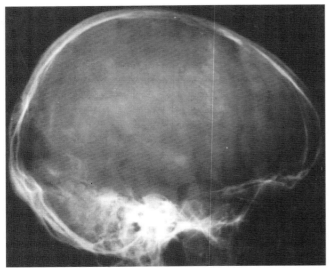

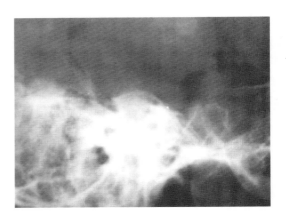

FIG 8—Fracture of the frontal bone affecting the anterior fossa floor (skull base). Subarachnoid air is seen in the subarachnoid space, anterior (adjacent to the dorsum sellae) and posterior to the brain stem (see enlargement).

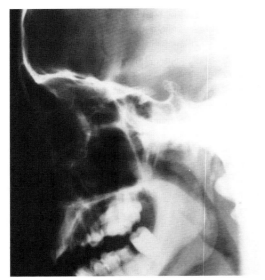

FIG 9—Basal skull fracture indicated by sphenoid and maxillary effusions. The fracture line extends into the lateral aspect of the frontal bone.

Check for intracranial air—Intracranial air (fig 8) appears as an area of relative translucency (blackness). An anterior aerocoele or air trapping around the brainstem means that the dura has been penetrated and that there is an open or compound injury which may require active management. In severe injuries intraventricular air can be identified.

Check the sinuses for air-fluid levels—Look at the sphenoid and frontal air sinuses to identify air-fluid levels. Lateral films in acute head injury are performed brow up with a horizontal *x* ray beam and air-fluid levels therefore appear as straight lines (fig 9). Air-fluid levels can be caused by a basal skull fracture, and this may be the only abnormality seen. Basal skull fractures are by definition "open" and can lead to intracranial infection.

Assessing other radiographs

Anteroposterior (fig 10)—The system of interpretation for the anteroposterior radiograph is similar to that for the lateral view. In addition to all the features examined in the lateral view look for pineal shift. If the pineal gland is calcified (60% of adults) shift can be assessed in a plain radiograph. Displacement greater than 2 mm suggests a space occupying lesion (haematoma, tumour) or oedema.

Half axial (Towne's)—This view should only be taken if cervical spine injury has been excluded (fig 5). Follow the same system as for the lateral radiograph but also look at the mastoid air cells when examining the bones.

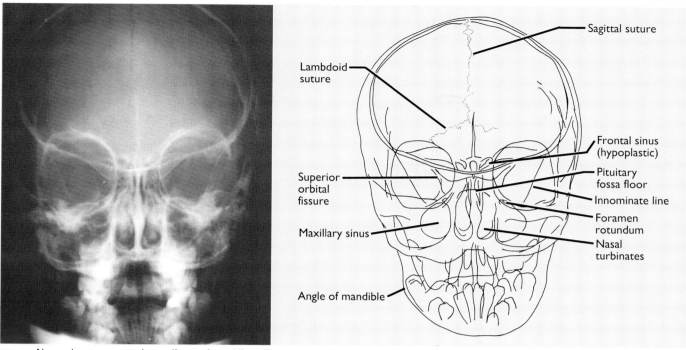

FIG 10—Normal anteroposterior radiograph and line diagram.

Catches to avoid

Characteristics of fractures, sutures, and vascular markings

Fractures

Straight translucent line

More radiolucent—fractures affect both tables

Most straight but can change direction suddenly

Sharply demarcated

Parallel margins—no tapering

May run across grooves or sutures

Sutures

Winding, serpiginous lines

Fine sclerotic or corticated margins, not sharply translucent

Typical anatomical site

Symmetrical

Vascular markings

Less translucent—affect inner table only

Not sharply demarcated

Meningeal grooves taper as they run peripherally

Branching pattern and symmetry

Diploetic venous channels are wide

The commonest diagnostic difficulty is deciding whether a translucent line is a fracture or a normal structure such as a suture or vascular marking. The metopic and mendosal (horizontal, accessory occipital suture) sutures occasionally persist into adult life and may cause confusion.

Causes of skull radiolucencies

Normal
Squamous temporal bone
Pacchionian granulations
Surgery

Air
Superficial—after scalp injury
Intracranial—seen in open fractures

Outer skull table
Rodent ulcer

Inner skull table
Slow growing tumours
Chronic subdural haematoma

Diffuse lesions
Metastases
Multiple myeloma
Paget's disease
Hyperparathyroidism

Causes of increased skull vault density

Generalised	*Multifocal*	*Localised*
Renal osteodystrophy	Sclerotic metastases	Foreign body
Fibrous dysplasia	Paget's disease	Hyperostosis frontalis interna
Fluorosis		Osteoma
Acromegaly		Meningioma
Drugs—for example, phenytoin		Hair bunch
Haemolytic anaemias		

Summary

Diagnostic quality

Bones
Sellae—size, erosion, shape
Cranium and base—fractures

Cartilage and joints
Sutures
Craniocervical region—C1/C2 fracture or subluxation, posterior nasal soft tissue

Soft tissues
Artefacts and foreign bodies
Intracranial air—anterior aerocoele, brain stem, intraventricular air
Sinus air-fluid levels—sphenoid, frontal, maxilla

Areas of reduced density are more common than sclerotic areas. There is a wide variation in the normal ossification of the calvaria, making differentiation of abnormalities difficult. Clinical history and examination are important in excluding many of the possible diagnoses.

MAXILLOFACIAL RADIOGRAPHS

D W Hodgkinson, R E Lloyd, P A Driscoll, D A Nicholson

> When the patient has a suspected cervical injury taking facial views can be dangerous because of the positioning that is required

This article deals with the problems facing non-specialist doctors requesting emergency radiographs of facial bones. An appropriate history and clinical examination will lead to suspicion of maxillofacial trauma and other pathology. We describe a systematic approach to requesting and interpreting maxillofacial views.

Important anatomy

Knowledge of the normal anatomy and radiological appearance of the skull is essential to interpreting radiographs of the face (see chapter on the skull).

> The radiological anatomy of the face revolves around the air space

The face can be divided into three areas: the upper third—area above the superior orbital margin; the middle third—area between the superior orbital margin above and the occlusal plane below; and the lower third—the lower jaw (mandible). Standard radiographic investigation of the face is described with reference to these three areas.

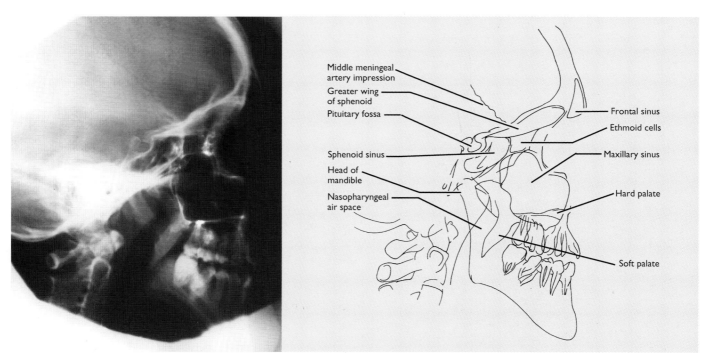

FIG 1—Lateral radiograph with line drawing showing radiological anatomy.

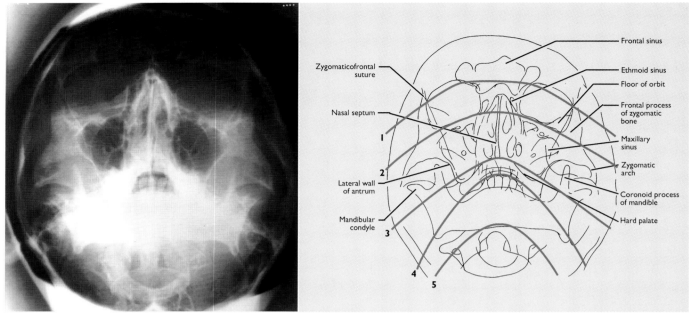

FIG 2—Occipitomental 45 radiograph with line drawing. The drawing also shows the five lines that should be traced when assessing the radiograph.

Mechanism of injury

In practice many injuries do not fit into the standard pattern of LeFort fractures. The classification is, however, still in general use for descriptive purposes

The mechanism of injury is an important aid to identifying the specific injury and any possible associated injuries. It can help decide which type of film to request and the urgency of the request. Isolated injuries to the maxillofacial skeleton commonly result from an assault. More severe injuries occur after high energy transfer (for example, road traffic accidents) and may be associated with injuries to the head, neck, chest, and other body regions.

Radiographic projections

Appropriate radiographic views for detecting trauma to maxillofacial regions

Anatomical site	Clinical findings	Radiographic view
Upper third: Nasoethmoid	Periorbital haematoma, epistaxis, displaced nasal bones, deviated nasal septum, cerebrospinal fluid rhinorrhoea, transverse cleft in glabellar region	Occipitofrontal and lateral
Orbits	Diplopia, enophthalmos, proptosis, restriction of ocular movements	Occipitofrontal and lateral
Middle third: Zygomatic complex	Periorbital oedema, haematoma, infraorbital anaesthesia, step deformities/flattening of the cheek	Occipitomental 45
Zygomatic arch	Depression over arch, restriction of mandibular movement	Submentovertical
Maxilla		Occipitomental 45
LeFort 1	Swelling of upper lip and cheek, mobile maxilla, teeth gagged posteriorly	Occipitomental 45 and lateral
LeFort 2 and 3	Facial oedema (severe in 3), periorbital haematoma, elongation of face (dished), mobile maxilla, teeth gagged posteriorly	Occipitomental 45 and lateral
Lower third: Mandible	Tenderness; bruising, swelling; bleeding from mouth or ear, or both; anaesthesia of lower lip; crepitus or mobile fracture, malocclusion or inability to close the teeth	Orthopantomogram and posteroanterior or Towne's, lateral oblique, and posteroanterior

Good quality, carefully positioned radiographs are required. This can be difficult to achieve in patients presenting to the emergency department (because of multiple injuries or alcohol intoxication). Poor quality and incorrectly positioned films must not be accepted. Radiology of a clinically suspected maxillofacial injury can often be delayed until the patient is more cooperative or good quality films can be taken.

The standard radiographic projections are listed below. Each projection provides only a limited amount of information, and several views are therefore required to assess an injury fully. The clinical findings should be used to determine the probable site of injury and dictate which views are most appropriate.

Radiological investigation of non-traumatic maxillofacial emergencies

Diagnosis	Clinical findings	Radiographic view
Periapical abscess	Facial pain or swelling	Orthopantomogram
Sinusitis	Facial pain, swelling, or tenderness	Occipitomental 45 (maxilla)
	Nasal discharge (maxilla)	Occipitofrontal (frontal/ethmoid)
Sialadenitis	Acute pain after eating	Posteroanterior
	Swelling of salivary gland	Lateral oblique

Occipitomental projection (45° and 30°)—These views are used to assess the maxilla (LeFort 1, 2, and 3 fractures), the zygomatic complex, and orbital floor (fig 2).

The lateral projection (fig 1) is used to assess all three parts of the face. It can be taken with the patient lying supine on the table with a portable unit (unlike the other projections).

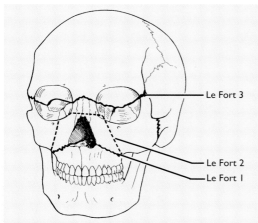

FIG 3—LeFort lines used for classifying fractures of the middle third of the face.

Occipitofrontal projection (25°)—This is used to assess the upper third of the face and orbits. The view projects the top edge of the petrous bones just below the infraorbital margins and thus shows the whole of the orbits.

The submentovertical projection is used to assess the zygomatic arch.

The orthopantomogram is used to assess the mandible. It is very informative but requires the cooperation of the patient because of the long exposure time. It is replacing the lateral oblique view as the best method of assessment.

Posteroanterior projection (10°)—This is used to assess the mandible.

Towne's view shows the ascending rami of the mandible and the condyles on each side.

Lateral oblique projection—These views are valuable for assessing the body of the mandible.

Nasal bones
A simple nasal bone fracture is diagnosed clinically, and routine radiography of the nasal bones is unnecessary. Trauma to the bridge of the nose may produce a nasoethmoid fracture. These patients usually have persistent epistaxis or cerebrospinal fluid rhinorrhoea, or both. This injury cannot be excluded by plain radiographs.

Temporomandibular joint projection
These specialised views should be requested only when specific information about the function of the joint is required. Non-specialists should not need to request or interpret these views. Fractures of the mandibular condyle are common and are diagnosed with other views. They rarely affect the temporomandibular joint except when the condyle and the glenoid fossa are fractured together in high energy trauma.

FIG 4—Submentovertical view showing a fractured left zygomatic arch.

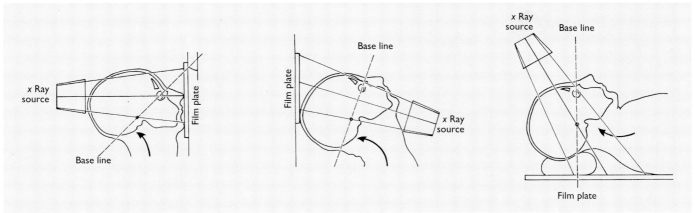

FIG 5—The positioning of the patient, the x ray source, and the film for (from left to right) the occipitomental 45, submentovertical, and Towne's views. The base line is the line drawn between the external auditory meatus and the orbit.

Radiological assessment of occipitomental view

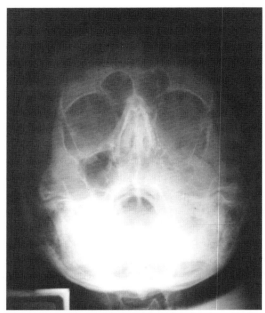

FIG 6—Occipitomental view showing fractured left zygoma. Note the increased size of the left orbit and opacification of the left maxillary sinus.

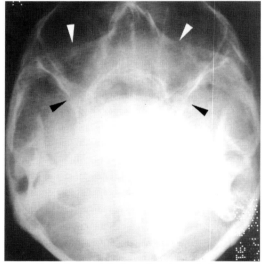

FIG 7—Occipitomental view showing a LeFort 2 fracture. Fractures are visible on both sides (arrows). The opacification of both maxillary sinuses and the general hazy appearance of the film is consistent with severe soft tissue swelling.

Radiographs should be interpreted by using the ABCs system.

Adequacy and quality of the radiograph

Start by identifying the name of the patient and the date on which the radiograph was taken. Then ensure that it is correctly centred by tracing a line that connects the nasal septum, the centre of the mandible, and the odontoid peg. This should be vertical, straight, and run through the centre of the film. Next look for rotation by tracing the outline of the orbits; they should be the same size and shape and the lateral walls should be of equal thickness and equidistant from the nasal septum. Another method of assessing rotation is to draw the imaginary Campbell line 2 (see below) and look for rotation of the orbits about a vertical and horizontal axis.

Alignment and bones

Figure 2 shows the five lines that should be traced when assessing the radiograph. They are known as Campbell's lines.

Line 1 joins the two zygomaticofrontal sutures. It runs along the superior orbital margin on each side and centrally across the region of the glabella. Check for any separation of the zygomaticofrontal suture and look at the integrity of the superior orbital margins.

Line 2 is traced from the zygomatic arch. It follows the zygomatic bone and continues along the inferior orbital margin across the frontal process of the maxilla and lateral wall of the nose through the septum. It then follows a similar course on the other side. Check the zygomatic arch for fractures then compare the transverse width of the frontal process of the maxilla and vertical dimensions of the zygomatic bones on the left and right side. Any asymmetry may indicate a fracture. Look for a break in continuity of the inferior orbital margin, particularly at the junction of the inner third and outer two thirds. A downward blow out fracture of the orbit may be seen (tear drop sign), but this is not a consistent feature in this injury.

Line 3 starts at the condyle of the mandible and traces across the mandibular notch and coronoid process to the lateral wall of the maxillary antrum. It continues through the medial wall of the antrum or lateral wall of the nose at the level of the nasal floor and then follows a similar course on the opposite side. Check the continuity of the maxillary antral walls and look for any depression of the orbital floor.

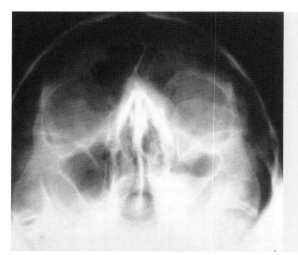

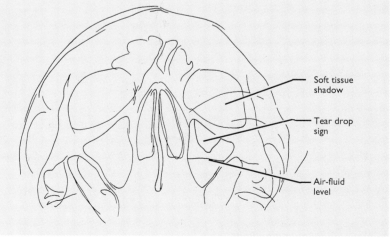

- Soft tissue shadow
- Tear drop sign
- Air-fluid level

FIG 8—Occipitomental view showing air-fluid level in the left maxillary sinus. Note tear drop sign projecting into the roof of the sinus (see line drawing). This is a feature of a downward blow out fracture of the orbit.

Any fluid level seen in a radiograph will depend on the orientation of the patient when the film was taken (erect or supine)

Indirect signs of maxillary fracture

● Soft tissue swelling
● Opacification of the maxillary sinus is usual in fractures which affect its wall and an air-fluid level is usually seen
● Soft tissue emphysema is a rare but useful sign. It provides positive evidence of a fracture of the nasal cavity or one of the paranasal sinuses. It may show as multiple small radiolucent areas in the soft tissues. Alternatively air may enter the orbit to outline the eyeball

Line 4 follows the occlusal curve of the upper and lower teeth. Check for evidence of mandibular fractures, although the definition may be poor and specific views are required for detailed assessment.

Line 5 traces the line of the lower border of the mandible. Check the continuity of this line.

Cartilages and joints

Look at the separation of the zygomaticofrontal suture located on line 1 above. Look for asymmetry between the two sides. The joint space should be smooth and thin, symmetrical along its length, and uninterrupted.

Sinuses

Check all the paranasal sinuses, in particular the frontal, maxillary, and ethmoid. Trace the outline of each sinus and look for any asymmetry between each side. Look for opacification of the sinus (complete or partial).

If a fluid level is suspected within the sinus the patient should have a brow up lateral projection taken. The orientation of the patient and therefore the air-fluid level will differ in the two views.

Discontinuity in the margins of the sinus indicates a fracture.

Soft tissue

Check the soft tissues by using a bright light. The soft tissue shadow from the line of the cheek can be seen traversing the orbit. If excessive swelling is present on one side the maxillary antrum on the same side may appear more radio-opaque. Look for a tear drop appearance in the top of the maxillary antrum. This may represent a blow out fracture of the orbital floor in the correct clinical context.

Check for foreign bodies within the soft tissues. Some objects (for example, glass) can be difficult to see without a bright light.

Important rules and diagnostic traps

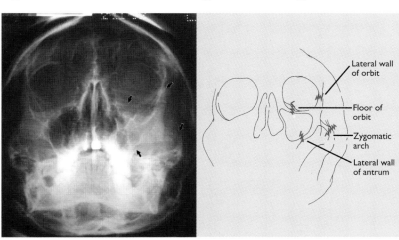

FIG 9—Occipitomental view showing a fractured zygomatic bone complex and line drawing showing disruption of all four legs of the stool (arrows).

Middle third of face

The zygomatic bone complex can be compared to a four legged stool with the legs being represented diagrammatically as: the floor of the orbit, the lateral wall of the orbit, the zygomatic arch, and the lateral wall of the antrum. The seat of a stool cannot be displaced without moving at least two of the legs. Likewise it is not possible to displace the zygomatic bone without fracturing two of the legs. Thus if one leg is thought to be fractured the other three must be checked.

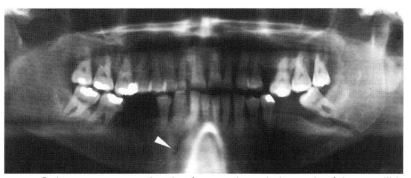

FIG 10—Orthopantomogram showing fracture through the angle of the mandible on the left side and a subtle fracture through the body on the right side (arrow).

Lower third of the face

When the mandible is injured it behaves as if it were a complete ring. This is because it is rigid and connected at each end of the skull by a firm joint. If one fracture of the mandible is found in the radiograph another fracture or dislocation may be present. Fractures of the angle of the mandible on one side are commonly associated with fractures through the mandibular condyle on the opposite side.

Common diagnostic traps in mandibular injuries

Summary

Adequacy

Alignment
    Check lines 1-5

Bones

Cartilage and joints
    Zygomaticofrontal suture

Sinuses
    Opacification
    Air-fluid levels

Soft tissue
    Swelling
    Foreign bodies

Normal anatomical structures can sometimes be mistaken for fractures. There are four common sites:
- Air in the oropharynx at the angle of the mandible. If checked carefully this line will extend beyond the outer cortex of the mandible
- Calcification or ossification of the stylohyoid ligament projecting over or just behind the ascending ramus
- The hyoid bone shown over the posterior part of the horizontal ramus
- The intervertebral spaces of the upper cervical vertebrae overlying the maxillae, simulating a LeFort 1 fracture, or over the mandibular symphysis, mimicking a dentoalveolar fracture.

Fractures of the mandible, particularly at the angle and the condyle, can appear undisplaced when seen in only one view. At least two views at right angles to each other are essential for full assessment—posteroanterior, Towne's, or lateral oblique.

The anterior mandible can be difficult to see in the orthopantomogram and lateral oblique projection because of superimposition of other structures. A lower occlusal view of the anterior mandible may therefore be useful in certain situations.

CERVICAL SPINE

P A Driscoll, R Ross, D A Nicholson

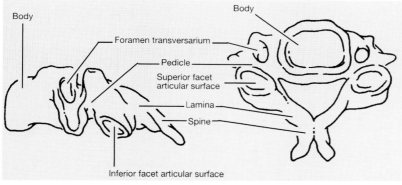

FIG 1—Lateral and aerial view of a cervical vertebra.

This chapter describes an effective system by which non-radiologists can analyse cervical spine radiographs and detect even the subtle signs caused by ligamental injuries. The system requires the clinician to be familiar with the basic anatomy of the cervical spine and understand how its structure can be damaged.

Anatomy

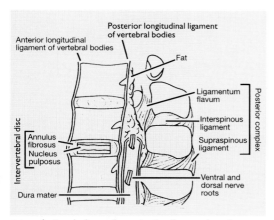

FIG 2—Lateral view of cervical column showing ligaments.

Stability and instability

A cervical injury is considered stable if controlled movements of the neck will not cause a neurological deficit. With an unstable injury, controlled movements of the neck are likely to produce or aggravate neurological damage

Steel's rule of three

The area demarcated by the bony ring of C1 is divided into thirds. One third is occupied by the odontoid, one third by an intervening potential space, and one third by the spinal cord

Adult

The cervical vertebrae are held together by a series of ligaments and paravertebral muscles, with the overall stability depending mainly on the integrity of the ligaments.

The anterior longitudinal ligament runs from the anterior arch of the atlas to the sacrum and is important in maintaining vertebral alignment. Similarly, the posterior longitudinal ligament connects the posterior aspect of the vertebral bodies. The posterior complex consists of the ligamentum flavum and the interspinous and supraspinous ligaments. The intertransverse ligament connects the transverse processes and forms the lateral column.

The spinal cord is contained within the spinal canal, where it is covered with three meningeal layers, blood vessels, and cerebrospinal fluid. The outer dural layer is separated from the bony canal by a space loosely filled with fat and blood vessels. The size of the extradural space varies with the relative diameters of the spinal cord and the spinal canal. As a consequence the body's ability to adapt to injuries that reduce the diameter of the canal depends on the site of the insult. For example, at the level of the axis (C2) the extradural space is large and therefore damage to the vertebral column in this area does not immediately impinge on the spinal cord. Disease processes or degenerative changes which reduce the size of the canal will also limit the vertebral column's ability to adapt to injury.

Developmental

Congenital malformations are common and should not be confused with traumatic lesions. They vary from minor defects to severe deformities such as fusion and hemivertebrae. In children normal developmental lines may be mistaken for fractures and lax ligaments for subluxation (see later).

Cervical spine
Mechanism of injury

The cervical spine is injured when it is subjected to a series of forces acting separately or in combination. A common area of important cervical injury is C1/C2 after impaction with the skull base. C5-C7 is a common site for disc degeneration, probably because of the reduced flexibility in this area.

Mechanisms of injury

Hyperflexion	Hyperextension and rotation
Hyperflexion and rotation	Compression
Hyperextension	

Hyperflexion can cause tears in the ligamental complex which widen the interspinous gap. It can also fracture the anterior superior corner of the vertebral body (flexion tear drop fracture) with posterior displacement of the rest of the fractured vertebra's body. This commonly occurs in the C5-C6 region.

In association with rotation, hyperflexion may produce tearing of the posterior ligamental complex, unifacet and bifacet dislocation, and avulsion of the spinous processes of C6-T1 (clay shoveller's fracture).

Injuries from hyperextension

General
Tearing of the anterior ligamental complex with widening of the anterior interdisc space
Tearing of the posterior ligaments allowing posterior displacement of the vertebral body
Avulsion fracture of anterior inferior corner of vertebral body (extension tear drop fracture)
Occasionally the spinous processes may be fractured

Atlas
Fracture of the laminae of C1
Avulsion fracture of the anterior arch of C1

Axis
Fracture through pars interarticularis of C2 (hangman's fracture)

The injuries resulting from hyperextension depend on where the force is exerted (box). Hyperextension and rotation can result in fracture of the lamina, pedicle, and the articular surface of vertebral bodies.

Compression can cause vertebral bodies to fracture with posterior displacement of bone fragments and soft tissue into the spinal canal.

Types of view

The lateral view is the routine radiograph for examining the cervical spine

---

Lateral, anteroposterior, and open mouth views are the routine radiographs of the cervical spine. Occasionally special projections, such as flexion-extension, swimmer's, and oblique views are required.

Interpretation of the lateral radiograph

A lateral cervical radiograph should show all the cervical vertebrae as well as the C7/T1 junction. Such a radiograph will detect 80-90% of cervical injuries.

ABCs approach to radiographic assessment

Alignment
Bones
Cartilage and joints
Soft tissue

Ligaments of the cervical spine cannot usually be seen in plain radiographs. Nevertheless, the effect of their disruption is often detectable. It is therefore important to follow a strict protocol when studying any radiograph so that subtle and multiple abnormalities are not missed. Therefore, once the adequacy of the film has been determined we advocate an ABCs approach.

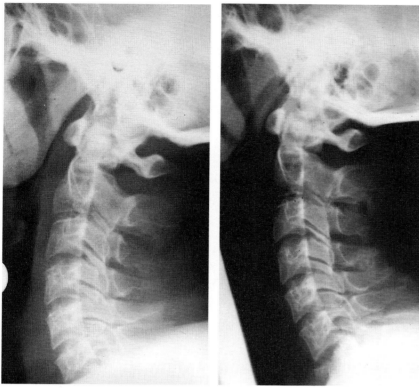

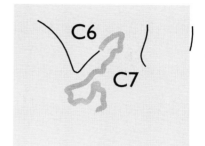

Check the adequacy and quality of the film

Count the number of vertebrae and make sure T1 is visible. Most diagnostic difficulties occur at the junctions (atlantoaxial and cervicothoracic). Most missed lesions occur at the cervicothoracic junction, usually because of an inadequate view.

FIG 3—Left: lateral radiograph showing no abnormality in the upper six cervical vertebrae; C7 and T1 are not seen. Right: the radiograph was repeated with the shoulders being pulled down, when a compression fracture of C7 became evident (line drawing).

Alignment

The anterior (1) and posterior (2) longitudinal lines should trace out a smooth lordotic curve from T1 to the base of the skull (fig 4). The intersection of line 3 is at the posterior rim of the foramen magnum. This spinolaminar line should also be a smooth curve, except at C2, where there can be a posterior displacement of up to 2 mm. Normally the tips of the spinous processes trace out a tight curve (4). The spinous processes tend to converge to a point behind the neck. Widening of the interspinous spaces is called divergence or "fanning." It is an abnormal sign and indicates that the posterior ligamental complex may be torn. A break in the contour of these lines may be due to facetal dislocation or a fractured vertebra. The commonest sites are C1/C2 and C6/C7.

> Anterior displacement greater than 3·5 mm in adults implies that the longitudinal ligaments are torn and, consequently, the cervical spine is unstable

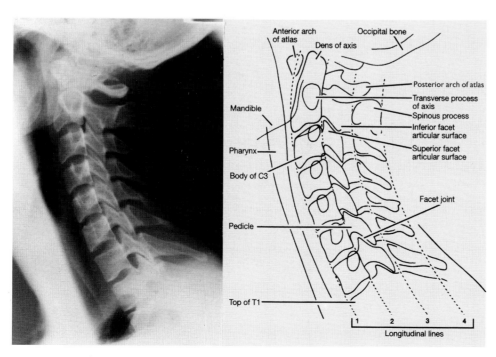

FIG 4—Lateral radiograph and line drawing with the four curves marked out. The anterior and posterior borders of the spinal canal are demarcated by the second and third longitudinal line.

Cervical spine

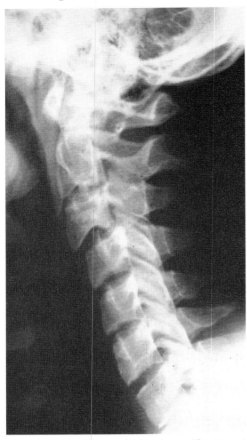

FIG 5—Lateral radiograph showing unifacet dislocation at C3/C4 with anterior displacement of C3 on C4. Below this level both facets are visible because of rotation. The increase in the soft tissue shadow is masked by the oesophagus starting at this level.

A unifacetal dislocation produces an anterior displacement of less than half of the width of a vertebral body. Inspection of the facet joint may show the inferior facet in the anterior position instead of the normal parallel articular surfaces with a joint space less than 2 mm. A more common sign is soft tissue swelling and rotation of the vertebrae so that both facet surfaces are seen in the lateral view—the bow tie sign. If unifacetal dislocation is suspected oblique views should be taken.

If the displacement is over 50% of the width of the vertebral body, bifacet dislocation is present. This is associated with fanning, narrowing of disc-disc space, and soft tissue swelling but no rotation (fig 6).

A simple loss of the cervical lordosis may be due to muscular spasm, age, previous injury, radiographic positioning, or a hard collar.

Bones

The cortical surface should be inspected first for steps, breaks, or abnormal angulations (figs 7-10). Start at the anterior inferior corner of the vertebra and then proceed in a clockwise fashion around the whole of the surface. Difficulty in following the cortical margins suggests overlapping of bone. This can result from a fracture or dislocation.

The rest of the vertebra is then inspected for alterations in the internal trabecular pattern, lucencies, and increases in density indicating a possible overlap of bone fragments (figs 9 and 10).

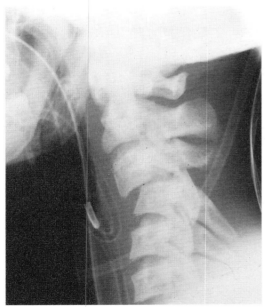

FIG 6—Lateral radiograph showing anterior slippage greater than 3·5 mm due to bifacet dislocation. Fanning of the spinous processes and narrowing of the disc space are visible. Soft tissue swelling is obscured by an endotracheal tube.

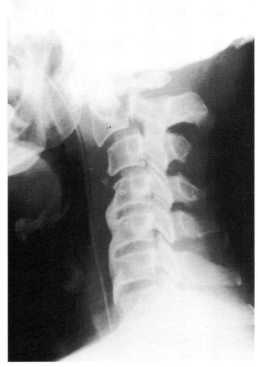

FIG 7—Lateral radiograph showing a hangman's fracture, anterior displacement of C2 on C3, opening of the posterior intervertebral disc space. Soft tissue swelling is present along with signs of ankylosing spondylitis.

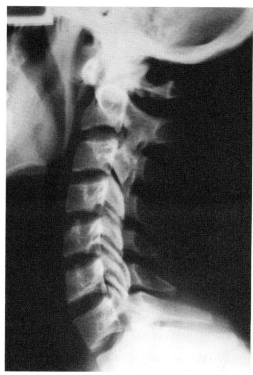

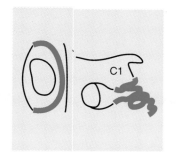

FIG 8—Lateral radiograph showing fracture of the lamina of C1 with anterior soft tissue swelling. The posterior border of the mandible should not be mistaken for the true soft tissue line.

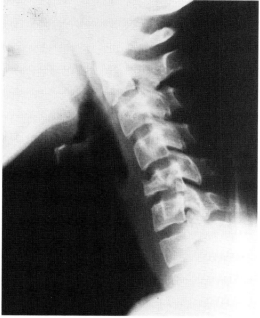

FIG 9—Lateral radiograph showing compression fracture of C5. The cortical surface is disrupted, the height of the vertebral body reduced, and trabecular pattern lost. Part of the posterior inferior corner of the vertebral body is projected backwards into the spinal canal.

A Jefferson fracture occurs when both the anterior and posterior aspects of the bony ring of C1 are compressed and fractured between the occipital condyles and C2. Open mouth and specialist views are used to distinguish this injury from isolated fractures of the lamina in C1 (fig 8). However, anterior soft tissue swelling usually indicates there is an anterior fracture as well. A third of these injuries are associated with fractures of C2.

Assessment of bones

Check each vertebra for deformity

Check the spinal canal

The heights of the anterior and posterior aspects of each vertebral body from C3 to T1 should be the same. A disparity of greater than 2 mm suggests a compression fracture (fig 9). A disparity greater than 25% can occur only if the posterior longitudinal ligament and posterior ligamental complexes are torn. It is therefore a sign of mechanical instability.

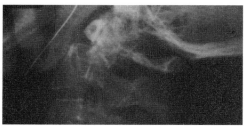

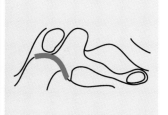

FIG 10—Lateral radiograph showing a fracture of the dens with posterior displacement into the spinal canal. This displacement causes the anterior longitudinal line to run along the front of the anterior part of C1, rather than along the front of the dens.

Never rush the examination of the lower vertebrae and, in particular, their spinous processes. These are prone to develop crush fractures after hyperextension and oblique avulsion fractures after hyperflexion with rotation.

The spinal canal should be over 13 mm wide from the posterior surface of the vertebral body to the spinolaminar line (fig 4). Narrowing of the canal can result from dislocations and compression fractures which displace segments of bone and soft tissue posteriorly (figs 9 and 10). Pre-existing disease and degeneration can also lead to narrowing of the canal.

Cartilage and joints

Check the disc spaces, facet joints, and interspinous gaps. The joint spaces should be similar to that at an adjacent vertebral level and the articulating surfaces should be parallel to one another. Calcification of these joints, associated ligaments, and intervertebral discs indicates ankylosing spondylitis (fig 7).

It is essential to assess the gap between the anterior surface of the dens and the posterior surface of the body of C1. This should be less than 3 mm in an adult and less than 5 mm in a child. Remember that the transverse atlantal ligament can rupture without there being any bony injury (for example, in rheumatoid arthritis).

Soft tissue shadows

Fractures to the cervical vertebrae produce haematomas that impinge on the black shadow of the oropharynx (figs 5, 8, 9). In children this gap can be wider because of crying, neck flexion, and pre-sphenoidal adenoidal enlargement. Pre-sphenoidal adenoidal enlargement increases the pre-vertebral soft tissue gap at C1/C2. Subtle fractures, ruptured ligaments, or haemorrhage may produce few radiological signs. However, displacement of the fat planes gives a clue that they are present. The fat planes can be seen as linear lucencies running parallel to the anterior longitudinal ligament. This sign is not usually affected by the presence of an endotracheal tube.

Several radiological features indicate possible cervical instability. However, until specialist advice is available it is safer to assume the lesion seen on the radiograph is unstable and to immobilise the neck accordingly.

In addition to the lateral cervical radiograph further views are commonly requested in trauma patients. These help detect another 10-15% of cervical abnormalities. However, the patient usually has to be moved to the radiology department for these radiographs to be taken. This should not be done until resuscitation is completed and the patient is stable from a respiratory and haemodynamic point of view. Radiographs should be assessed by usng the ABCs system described for the lateral view.

Radiological features of possible cervical instability

Facet joint overriding

Facet joint widening

Interspinous fanning

Greater than 25% compression of vertebral body

Over 10° angulations between vertebral bodies

Over 3·5 mm anterior vertebral body overriding with fracture

Tear drop fracture (flexion and extension)

Hyperextension fracture

Hyperextension fracture-dislocation

Jefferson fracture

Hangman's fracture

Soft tissue dimensions

Adults

C1-C4/5	7 mm
C4/5-T1	21 mm (one vertebral body)

Children

C4/5-T1	14 mm

Anteroposterior cervical radiograph

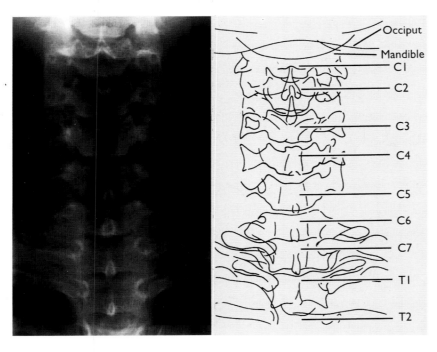

FIG 11—Anteroposterior radiograph and line diagram showing C1-T2. The spinous processes are aligned normally.

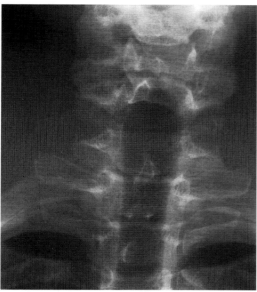

FIG 12—Anteroposterior radiograph showing unifacet dislocation of C6 (arrow). The spinous process of C6 is rotated to the right compared with the spinous processes of C5, C7, T1. The C6/7 intervertebral space is widened.

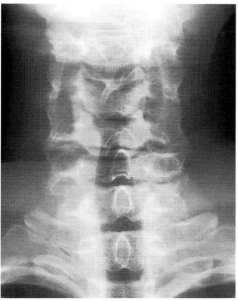

FIG 13—Anteroposterior radiograph showing crush fracture of C6. The height of C6 is reduced.

Adequacy

Ensure that T1 to C3 are visible. The mandible and occiput overlie C1-3 in this projection and may obscure them from view.

Alignment

Check alignment of spinous processes. Malalignment may indicate a unifacet dislocation or a fracture of the lateral articular surface. These injuries cause the spinous processes to rotate to the side of the injury.

Bones

The cortical surface of each vertebra must be inspected for steps, breaks, or abnormal angulations. Start at the right inferior corner of the vertebra and then proceed clockwise around the whole of the surface. Vertebral bodies should be rectangular. A careful inspection will reveal any compression, vertical fissures, and steps in the end plates.

The rest of the vertebra is then inspected for alterations in the internal trabecular pattern, lucencies, and increases in density indicating a possible overlap of bone fragments.

Cartilage and joints

Check each intervertebral joint space. The height should be similar to that found at adjacent vertebral levels and the articulating surfaces should be parallel to one another (compare figs 11 and 13).

Soft tissues

The paravertebral tissue must be assessed. Disruption of the normal air shadow may indicate an underlying fracture or dislocation.

Open mouth view

Adequacy

Check that the open mouth view shows the C1/C2 articulation.

Alignment

Check the alignment of the odontoid peg and C1/C2. Normally the dens and spinous process of C2 are in the same vertical line as are the lateral borders of C1 and C2. In adults there is normally less than 2 mm lateral overriding between C1 and C2 and the distances between the lateral masses of the atlas and the odontoid peg (dens) should be symmetrical.

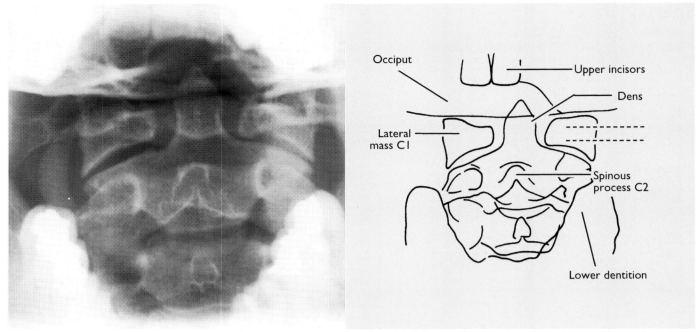

FIG 14—Left: Open mouth view. The dens and the spinous process of C2 are aligned normally, there is no lateral overriding of C1 on C2, and the dens is symmetrically placed between the two lateral masses of C1. Notice the artefact created by the occiput overlying the dens. This can be mistaken for a fracture. Right: Line diagram of the radiograph.

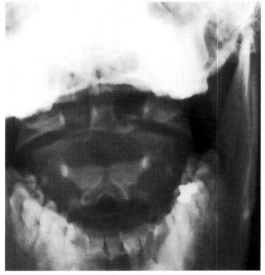

FIG 15—Open mouth view showing a Jefferson fracture. Both lateral masses of C1 are overlapping the lateral borders of C2. Notice the artefact created by the incisors overlapping the dens.

Jefferson fractures are often seen clearly in this view. Rotatory subluxation of the odontoid in children is also best shown by the open mouth view. Up to the age of 8, incomplete ossification of the dens and ligamental laxity allows up to two thirds of the anterior arch of C1 to lie above the odontoid peg.

Bones

Check the odontoid peg and examine the dens carefully. Fractures can occur in the peg itself (type 1) or at its base (type 2) or can extend into the body of C2 (type 3). Type 2 fractures are the commonest and lead to instability of the cervical spine. The dark shadow of the overlying teeth, the occiput, or the epiphyseal plate is often mistaken for fracture (fig 14). The epiphysis is V-shaped and should have fused by 12 years of age. Non-union of this secondary ossification centre leads to formation of an os odontoideum, which appears with a characteristic smooth convex border at the tip of the dens.

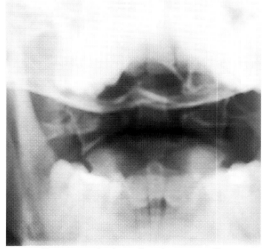

FIG 16—Open mouth view showing a type 2 fracture of the dens.

Cartilage and joints

Check the joint space between C1 and C2. The articulating surfaces should be parallel to one another.

Soft tissues

The paravertebral tissue should be inspected, although soft tissue shadows are not usually evident in this view.

Special views

Swimmer's view

The swimmer's view should be requested if C7/T1 cannot be seen on the normal lateral cervical radiograph. The film looks strange because it is showing a focused oblique view of the C7/T1 junction. However, the feature to concentrate on is the anterior alignment of the vertebral bodies.

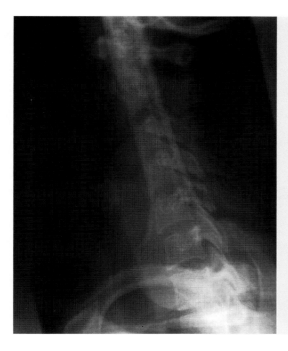
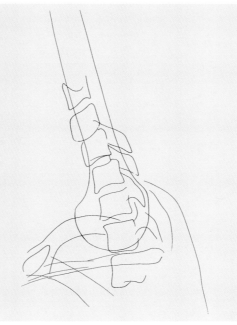

FIG 17—Swimmer's view and line diagram showing C5-T1. The anterior longitudinal line is broken because of the forward slip of C7 on T1. This resulted from a unifacet dislocation. A normal air shadow caused by the trachea is clearly seen.

Oblique view

This gives a good view of the intervertebral formina and the facet joints. It is usually requested by specialists when a unifacet dislocation is suspected from the routine films.

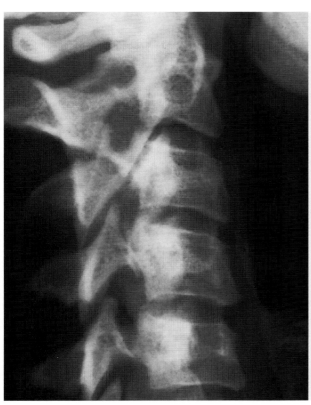
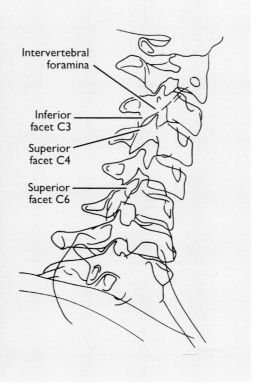

Intervertebral foramina

Inferior facet C3

Superior facet C4

Superior facet C6

FIG 18—Oblique view and line diagram of the cervical column. The superior facet of C6 is fractured and displaced into the intervertebral foramina. This view clearly shows the facet joints and intervertebral foramina.

Cervical spine

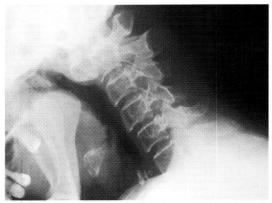

FIG 19—Lateral radiograph showing a flexion view of the cervical spine. The standard view appeared normal, but on flexion C1 subluxates forward and an abnormally wide gap develops between the dens and the anterior arch of C1.

Flexion and extension views

These radiographs are taken when a specialist has reviewed the standard radiographs and considers there is cervical malalignment with no corresponding significant soft tissue swelling, subluxation, or widening of facet joints. All neck movements must be carried out by a doctor and the patient must be conscious. This allows the procedure to be stopped immediately any pain or neurological symptoms develop.

These views are modified lateral radiographs and should be examined using the ABCs system.

Catches to avoid

> The absence of radiological abnormality reduces the chances of spinal injury but does not exclude it. About 8% of patients have injuries to the cervical spine in more than one place and 15% of patients with cervical injury also have a thoracolumbar injury

Make sure all seven cervical vertebrae and the C7/T1 junction are visible. The spinous processes may not be clear. If you suspect an injury obtain a further view. Do not forget to examine the soft tissue shadows; these may be the only clues to an underlying fracture.

Physiological subluxation of the bodies of C2 on C3 (seen in a quarter of cases) and C3 on C4 (seen in 15% of cases) occurs up to 8 years of age. However, the posterior spinal line is maintained.

Artefactual shadows can sometimes cause confusion. In the open mouth view the vertical cleft between the upper two incisor teeth may be mistaken for a vertical fracture of the peg.

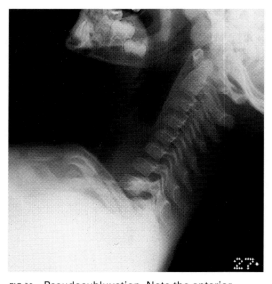

FIG 20—Pseudosubluxation. Note the anterior subluxation of the bodies of C2 on C3 and C3 on C4. It can be distinguished from true subluxation by noting that no break is present in the vertical line running through the spinolaminar junction.

> **Summary**
>
> *Adequacy and quality*
> Ensure that the vertebrae C1-C7 and the C7/T1 junction are visible
>
> *Alignment*
> Assess the contours of the cervical spine and appendages
>
> *Bones*
> Check each vertebra for shape, height, and fractures
> Check the shape of the odontoid peg
> Check spinal canal size
>
> *Cartilage and joints*
> Check the intervertebral disc spaces
> Check the facet joints
> Check the interspinous distance
> Check the C1/C2 distance
>
> *Soft tissues*
> Check the precervical and paracervical spaces

THORACIC AND LUMBAR SPINE

P A Driscoll, D A Nicholson, R Ross

> All injuries of vertebral column should be treated as unstable until a specialist advises otherwise.

This chapter describes a system by which non-radiologists can analyse the common radiographs taken of the thoracic and lumbar spine and the sacrolumbar junction. The system requires knowledge of the basic anatomy of the vertebral column and an understanding of how it can be injured.

Important anatomical considerations

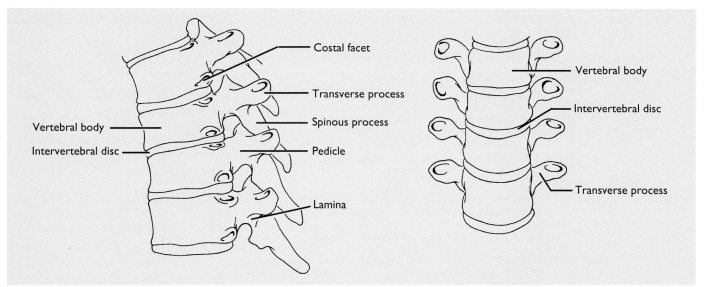

FIG 1—Left: Line diagram showing lateral view of the thoracic vertebral column. Right: Line diagram showing anteroposterior view of the thoracic vertebral column.

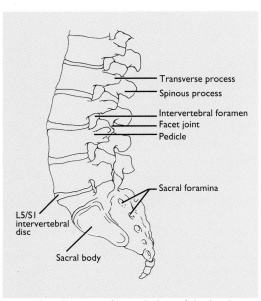

FIG 2—Line diagram of lateral view of the lumbar vertebral column.

This part of the vertebral column is more stable than the cervical spine because of the nature of the ligaments, intervertebral discs, facet joint alignment, paravertebral muscles, and the upper eight ribs (thoracic). The ligaments are the most important stabilising feature.

In view of these stabilising features vertebral disruption in the thoracic or lumbar area occurs only when a large force has been applied—usually with rotation. This is particularly true in the case of the thoracic vertebrae, which have additional support from the ribs.

Nevertheless, the vertebral column can be damaged, especially where the curvature of the spine alters. The mechanical stresses which result from the change in direction at the thoracolumbar junction (T11-L2) or sacrolumbar junction are amplified by the differing mobility above and below the junction. These areas are therefore common sites of injury when the vertebral column is subjected to abnormal forces.

Thoracic and lumbar spine

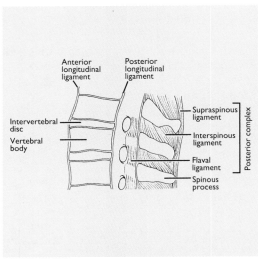

FIG 3—Line diagram of important ligaments in the thoracolumbar spine.

Two thirds of fractures in the thoracic and lumbar region occur between T12 and L2

Spinal canal

The spinal cord and its meningeal coverings run down the spinal canal to the level of the L1/2 disc (adult) or L2/3 vertebrae (new born). Between the bony canal and the dura mater is a potential space that is normally filled with extradural fat and blood vessels. The size of the space varies with the region of the vertebral column and the presence of degenerative disease. For example, in the thoracic area the space is small because the spinal cord is wide. This region therefore has a limited capacity to adapt to injuries that impinge on the spinal canal.

Developmental

Each vertebra ossifies from three centres, any of which can fail to fuse. This gives rise to deformities such as hemivertebra. Spina bifida occulta is caused by a failure of the dorsal parts of the vertebrae to fuse and usually occurs in the sacrolumbar region.

Lumbarisation is incomplete fusion of the upper sacral vertebrae. In sacralisation, the vertebra of L5 is partly or completely fused with the ala (top) of the sacrum.

Mechanism of injury

Common mechanisms of injury

Hyperflexion—Usually occurs at T12-L2 in adults and T4/5 in children. The posterior structures are stretched and the anterior ones compressed. This force usually causes a wedge fracture. If the person is constrained by a lap belt, however, a horizontal fracture through the body, pedicle, and posterior vertebra is seen (Chance fracture)

Shearing—The vertebra is slid anteriorly or posteriorly with respect to the one below. All the intervertebral ligaments can be torn and displacement may be up to 25%

Hyperextension tears the longitudinal ligaments and widens the anterior disc space. It can be associated with avulsion fracture of the anterior superior vertebral corner

Axial compression squeezes the vertebral bodies of T4-L5 together. The intervertebral disc explodes under excessive force, disrupting the longitudinal ligaments

The thoracic and lumbar regions of the vertebral column are damaged by forces that produce extreme movements such as hyperflexion, hyperextension, and axial compression. These forces are usually modified by other forces which cause rotation, distraction, and lateral flexion to occur at the same time. The commonest cause of fractures of the thoracic lumbar spine is hyperflexion with rotation resulting from falls, direct trauma, or road traffic accidents.

Radiological interpretation of lateral view

Types of view

Lateral

Anteroposterior

Sacrolumbar junction

Oblique

ABCs system of radiographic interpretation

Alignment
Bones
Cartilage and joints
Soft tissue

After the patient's name, the date, and the adequacy of the radiographs have been determined the films should be examined by using the ABCs system.

Check the adequacy and quality of the film

Count the vertebrae and make sure that all five lumbar vertebrae, the sacrolumbar junction, and the thoracic vertebrae can be seen clearly.

Alignment

The anterior and posterior longitudinal lines should be smooth curves which change direction at the thoracolumbar and sacrolumbar junctions. In the lumbar region there should also be a smooth curve through the facet joints. This is difficult to see in the thoracic region because of the overlying ribs. At the sacrolumbar junction the upper surface of the sacrum slopes downwards.

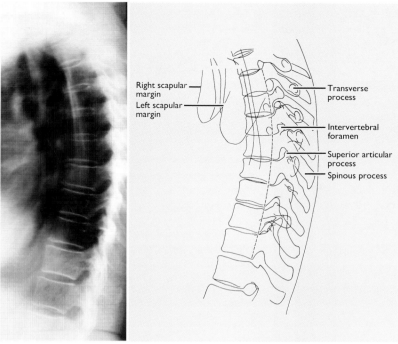

FIG 4—Lateral radiograph and line diagram showing the normal alignment of the thoracic vertebrae.

Bones

Each vertebra must be assessed individually. First look at the cortical surface for steps, breaks, or abnormal angulations. Start at the anterior inferior corner of the vertebra and proceed clockwise around the whole of the surface. If you cannot trace out the cortical margins there is usually an overlap of bone. In the upper thoracic region the facet joints, spinous processes, and transverse processes normally cannot be seen because of the alignment of the facet joints and overlying ribs, scapula, and soft tissues. Elsewhere in the vertebral column, loss of cortical margin is commonly caused by a fracture or dislocation.

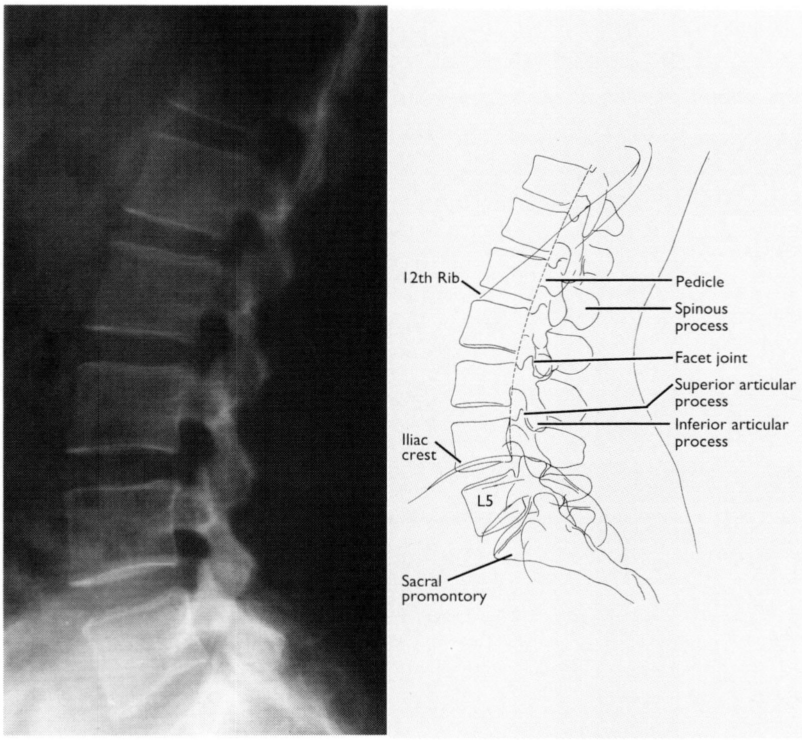

Look at the rest of each vertebra for alterations in the internal trabecular pattern, lucencies, and increases in density. A discrepancy ≥ 2 mm between the anterior and posterior height of the vertebral body indicates a fracture except at T11-L1, where these dimensions can exist normally. A 50% discrepancy is always abnormal and suggests serious ligamental damage (fig 6). This injury is often associated with soft tissue swelling and, in extreme situations, subluxation of the facet joint and widening of the interspinous gaps.

FIG 5—Lateral radiograph and line diagram showing the normal alignment of the lumbar vertebrae and the sacrolumbar junction.

A Chance fracture can usually be seen in the lateral view (fig 7). The fracture line may extend into the pedicles and lamina and, sometimes, an increase in posterior vertebral height with widening of the posterior disc space is seen.

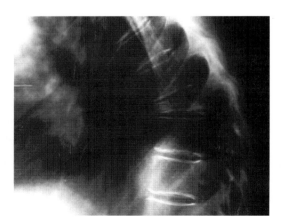

FIG 6—Lateral radiograph of the thoracic vertebrae showing a wedge fracture which is greater than 50% of the vertebral height. The adjacent intervertebral disc spaces are narrowed.

Reduced height of both the anterior and the posterior surfaces relative to the height in the adjacent vertebra indicates an axial compression force (fig 8). This is commonly associated with soft tissue swelling, anterior wedging, vertical fractures of the spinolaminar junctions, and posterior displacement of fragments into the spinal canal.

Thoracic and lumbar spine

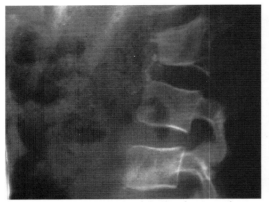

FIG 7—Lateral radiograph of the lumbar vertebrae showing a Chance fracture of the vertebral body of L2. The posterior vertebral body height is greater than the anterior surface.

Effect of forces on joint space

Hyperflexion—anterior narrowing

Hyperextension—widening

Axial compression—total disruption

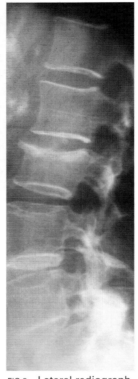

FIG 8—Lateral radiograph of the lumbar vertebrae showing an axial compression fracture with disruption of the superior articular surface of L3.

Hyperextension injuries can cause widening of the anterior disc space, fracturing of the laminae and spinous processes, and posterior displacement of bony fragments. Fractures of the transverse and spinous processes can occur in isolation after direct trauma but they are usually associated with other fractures.

Cartilage and joints

Check each intervertebral disc. The discs should be similar and even throughout, with their height increasing progressively down the spine to L4/L5. The disc at L5/S1 is usually narrower than that at L4/L5.

Check the facet joint for alignment. Unilateral or bilateral dislocation of the facet can occur in the lumbar region after trauma but only in association with severe damage to the vertebral body.

Soft tissue

Check the soft tissue shadows around the vertebral column. Disruption of shadows indicates there may be an underlying bony or ligamental injury.

Anteroposterior view

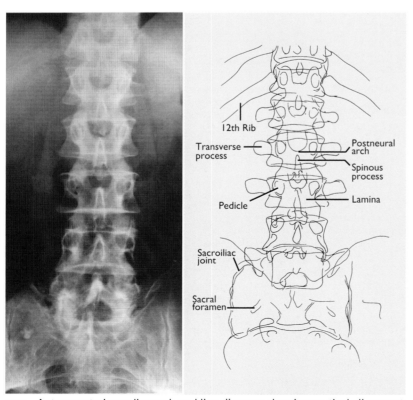

FIG 9—Anteroposterior radiograph and line diagram showing vertical alignment of the spinous processes and the gradual increase in width of the lumbar vertebrae and the interpedicular distance.

The anteroposterior radiograph should be examined with the same system described for the lateral radiograph.

Alignment

Check the vertical alignment of the spinous processes. The width of the vertebrae and the interpedicular distance increase progressively down the vertebral column (fig 9).

Malalignment may indicate a fracture of the lateral articular surface. In these cases the spinous processes rotate to the side of the injury.

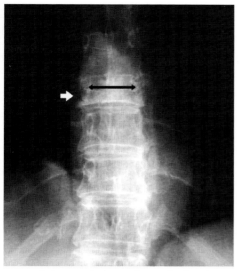

FIG 10—Anteroposterior radiograph showing a crush fracture of T8 with widening of the interpedicular space.

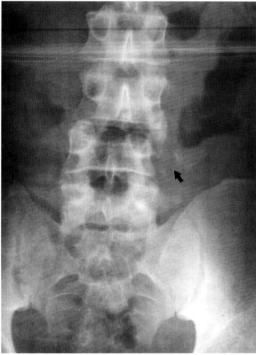

FIG 11—Anteroposterior radiograph of the lumbar vertebrae showing a crush fracture of L4 with rotation of the spinous processes of L4 and L5 to the right. There is also a fracture of the transverse process of L4.

Special views

Special views are rarely required in emergencies. They should be requested only after resuscitation has been completed and after consultation with the specialist in charge of the long term management of the patient

Bones

Assess each vertebra, starting with the cortical margin and finishing with underlying trabecular bone. The superior and inferior surfaces of the vertebral body should be parallel. A compression injury, which causes bursting of the vertebral body, can be detected in the anteroposterior view. In these cases there is loss of trabecular pattern, overlapping of bone fragments, and widening of the interpedicular distance (fig 10). Interpedicular widening usually denotes serious bone damage and ligamental disruption.

Examine the upper thoracic vertebrae carefully because they cannot be seen clearly in the lateral radiograph. Occasionally lateral wedging of the vertebral bodies occurs due to lateral flexion and rotation.

The transverse processes must also be inspected carefully. Depending on the quality of the film you may need a bright light to assess the tips of the processes in the lumbar region (fig 11). Fractures in this area usually result from muscular contraction. However, they can be caused by direct trauma and so damage to the overlying viscera should be looked for. Features of the sacrum seen in the anteroposterior radiograph are covered in the chapter on the pelvis.

Cartilage and joints

The intervertebral disc space should be examined as in the lateral view. The facet joints overlying each vertebral body should have a similar shape and position.

Soft tissue

Changes in the soft tissue after fracture of the upper thoracic vertebrae can mimic a ruptured thoracic aorta. Changes are best seen in a plain anteroposterior view of the chest. The psoas shadow and its importance is described in the chapter on the abdomen.

Soft tissue signs resulting from fractures of upper thoracic vertebrae

Left apical capping
Paravertebral haematoma
Mediastinal widening (80% of cases)

Oblique views enable assessment of the intervertebral foramina, the pedicles, and the facet joints. They may also be requested when spondylolithesis or unifacet dislocation is suspected.

Sternum and ribs—Injury leading to damage of the upper eight thoracic vertebrae can also fracture the sternum or ribs. This increases the chances of the thoracic injury being unstable. Radiographs of the sternum and relevant ribs should be taken.

Computed tomography enables specialists to assess the extent of the injury accurately. For example, it is routinely done to determine the degree of cord compression and the position of the bone fragments after axial compression.

Catches to avoid

Summary

Adequacy and quality
Ensure that all the vertebrae are visible

Alignment
Assess the contours of the thoracic and lumbar regions
Assess the change in curvature at the thoracolumbar and sacrolumbar junctions

Bones
Check each vertebra for shape, height, fractures, and interpedicular distance

Cartilage and joints
Check the facet joints
Check the intervertebral disc spaces
Check the interspinous distance

Soft tissue
Check the paravertebral spaces

The upper thoracic vertebral column is difficult to see in the lateral view because of the overlying shoulder girdle. Computed tomography should be requested if injury to this area is strongly suspected.

Make sure that all the required vertebrae are seen. Ask for further views if necessary.

The forces required to fracture the upper thoracic vertebrae are so great that there are often injuries elsewhere in the vertebral column.

Half of the patients with compression fractures have injuries elsewhere in the vertebral column.

Abnormal fusion during development can produce deformities such as symptomless joints that can be mistaken for fractures. In these cases the breaks in the cortex usually have a defined sclerotic margin.

TEN COMMANDMENTS OF EMERGENCY RADIOLOGY

R Touquet, P A Driscoll, D A Nicholson

Inexperienced and tired doctors can easily make mistakes, especially when requesting and interpreting emergency radiographs. To minimise the chances and consequences of such errors, this chapter describes ten general principles.

Command 1: take a history and examine the patient before requesting radiographs

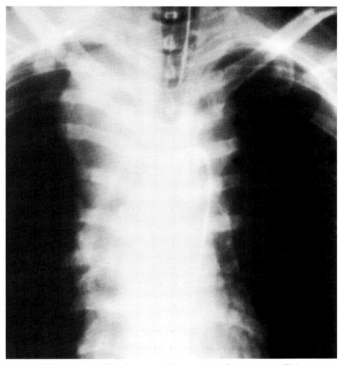

FIG 1—Widened mediastinum with rupture of the aorta. This condition was suspected as the patient's chest was subjected to a rapid deceleration injury in a road traffic accident.

A thorough history and examination enables you to establish the mechanism of injury and therefore decide what abnormalities are likely. The appropriate radiographs can then be requested and systematically interpreted (fig 1).

Knowledge of the mechanism of injury also helps determine the likely pattern of injuries and any associated pathology. Examine all areas that are suspected to have been affected so that injuries are not missed. Additional radiographs of areas away from the site of the injury may therefore be needed.

> **Injuries associated with particular conditions**
> - Colles' fracture with concomitant fracture of radial head
> - Ankle injury with fracture of the styloid process of the fifth metatarsal
> - Pain in the knee from slipped femoral epiphysis
> - Pain in arm from nerve root entrapment in the neck

Command 2: treat the patient, not the radiograph

> **Examples of conditions whose diagnosis relies mainly on clinical findings**
> - Scaphoid fracture
> - Base of skull fracture
> - Epiphyseal injuries—for example Salter-Harris type I injury without shift

Conditions such as a tension pneumothorax are life threatening and require immediate treatment before a confirmatory radiograph is taken. Furthermore, the diagnosis of certain injuries depends on the clinical findings. In such cases the radiograph helps to confirm the diagnosis but does not prevent the appropriate treatment being carried out when no radiological abnormality can be identified.

Command 3: never look at a radiograph without seeing the patient

When receiving a patient **do not** perpetuate any diagnostic errors

Irrespective of grade or experience you should always insist on seeing the patient when asked to interpret a radiograph. This is particularly important when patients are transferred to another medical team or handed over at the end of a shift in the accident and emergency department. Although all radiographs should be interpreted systematically, seeing the patient will enable the radiological findings to be correlated with the clinical examination and so help reduce the chances of missing an abnormality or perpetuating an error already made.

Command 4: always review the radiographs in appropriate settings

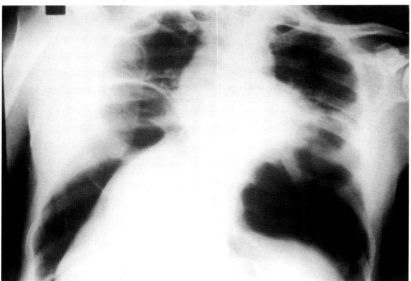

Films should ideally be assessed in a dark room with a proper viewing box and an additional bright light for interpreting low density areas such as the soft tissues. Avoid standing or sitting too close to the radiograph. Studying radiographs close up in a well lit room with many distractions increases the chances of missing abnormalities (fig 2).

FIG 2—Distraction can cause a clinician to detect only the severe abnormality (the pneumoperitoneum) and miss the subtle pneumothorax.

Command 5: view every film, the whole film, and the film as a whole

The AABCs system for interpreting radiographs
Adequacy
Alignment
Bones
Cartilage and joints
Soft tissues

A common mistake is to focus immediately on severe abnormalities or particular areas of the radiograph. This can mean that the whole film is not inspected and consequently additional abnormalities are missed. Such mistakes can be avoided by always using a system for inspecting the whole radiograph. The systems for reading each emergency radiograph have been described in the appropriate chapters of this book. In general they follow the AABCs approach, but this is modified for regions such as the chest and abdomen.

Command 6: re-examine the patient when the radiograph does not show the expected findings

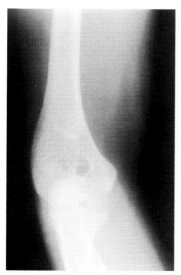
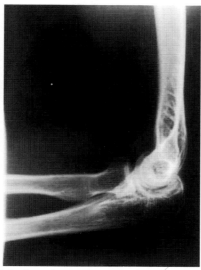
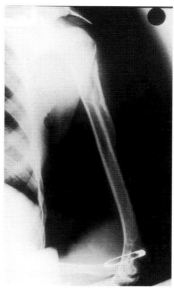

FIG 3—(Left) Normal radiograph of a left elbow in a patient who had fallen down the stairs and attended the accident department in great pain holding her arm. (Right) Radiograph of the same patient taken the next day when she reattended having been previously reassured and sent home. She had a fractured proximal left humerus with a butterfly fragment.

When a radiograph does not show what you expected, or shows something inconsistent with the clinical findings, it is essential to check that the correct part and side of the body has been radiographed and that the site of injury has been appropriately identified (fig 3). Occasionally special views will be required to show an abnormality if there is clinical suspicion of a particular injury.

Command 7: remember the rule of two

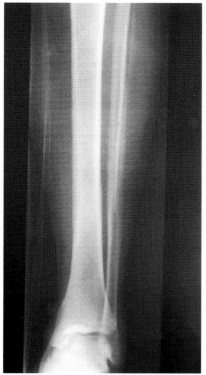
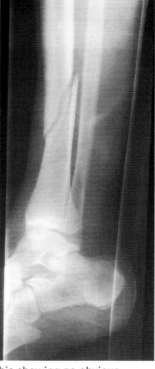

FIG 4—(Left) Anteroposterior view of right tibia showing no obvious abnormality. (Right) The lateral view of the same region shows an obvious fracture.

The rule of two is easy to remember and follow. It is particularly helpful if you are inexperienced.

Two views—A fracture may be visible in only one view because of its alignment (fig 4). Consequently two views at right angles should be taken.

Two joints—Because of the risk of associated dislocation or subluxation always include the joint at either end of long bones when a fracture is suspected (fig 5).

Two sides—Comparison of the normal and injured sides in children will help detect subtle epiphyseal injuries. Variation in the alignment of joints is important to note because it may obscure abnormalities. Comparing one side with the other will help you spot these variations (fig 6).

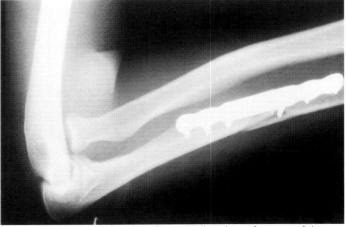

FIG 5—Lateral view of the right forearm showing a fracture of the ulna (plated) with a corresponding dislocation of the radial head.

Two radiographs—Certain fractures, such as those of the neck of the talus, are difficult to detect. However, when a radiograph is compared with a film of a normal neck the fracture becomes easier to see.

Two occasions—The natural course of certain conditions may mean that radiography needs to be repeated at a later date to show the abnormality—for example, the stress fracture.

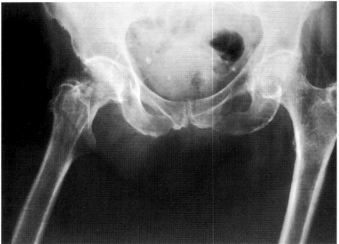
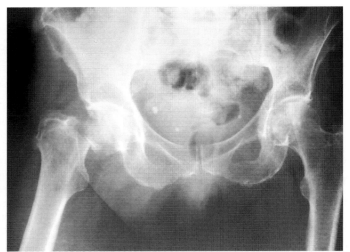

FIG 6—(Left) Anteroposterior view of the pelvis. Note the internal rotation of right femur with the greater trochanter obscuring the neck of the femur. (Right) A repeat radiograph after the right femur had been placed into the same position as the left clearly shows a fracture of the neck of the right femur.

Command 8: take radiographs before and after procedures

After removing a foreign body it is important to take a follow up radiograph to determine if any pieces remain (fig 7). The patient must be informed if a foreign body cannot be found or if it is inappropriate to remove it. In both cases a definitive note must be made in the records. Similarly, repeat radiographs are required after reductions of dislocations and fractures to confirm the new position is satisfactory.

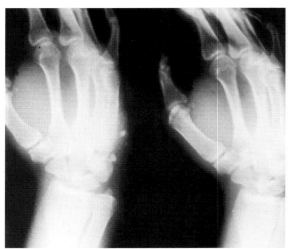
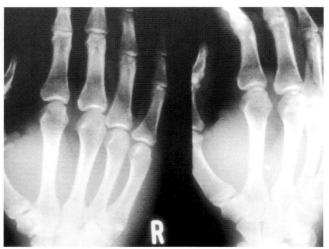

FIG 7—Pieces of glass in the hand before (left) and after (right) attempted removal.

Command 9: if a radiograph does not look quite right ask and listen

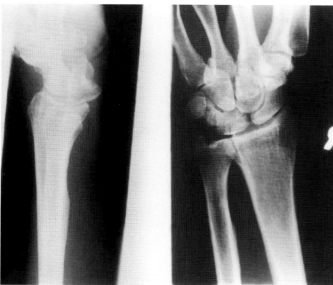

FIG 8—Anteroposterior and lateral view of the carpus showing a dislocated lunate.

Inexperienced doctors are likely to come across injuries that they have never seen before. You will often notice that the radiograph does not look quite right but not be able to determine the correct diagnosis (fig 8). When this occurs it is important to seek senior advice.

Many departments operate a "red dot" system, in which the radiographer flags up an abnormality. Though this is helpful, the absence of a red dot does not necessarily mean there is no abnormality. It is important to remember this because the final responsibility lies with the doctor in charge of the case not with the radiographer.

Command 10: ensure you are protected by fail safe mechanisms

Quality control system for interpreting radiographs

- After reviewing the radiographs the doctor should record the radiological diagnosis on the request card

- All emergency radiographs must be reviewed by a radiologist, and the report returned within 72 hours. (Many would now advocate immediate reporting)

- The radiologist should record at the end of his report whether he or she agrees or disagrees, with the doctor's diagnosis

- All radiographs need to be reviewed if the report states disagree. The radiologist should telephone the department at once if a serious injury has been missed

---

Radiological diagnoses will sometimes be missed by all grades of staff. The consultant is responsible for setting up systems to minimise the effect of these clinical errors. To miss an injury radiologically may not be negligent but not to have systems in place to cater for that eventuality is. These fail safe mechanisms must be audited regularly, and adequate facilities, education, and staffing levels need to be provided.[1]

1 Touquet R, Fothergill J, Harris N. Accident and emergency departments: the speciality of accident and emergency medicine. In: Powers M, Harris N, eds. *Medical negligence*. 2nd ed. London: Butterworths, 1994.

INDEX

Index

Index